Pediatric Interviewing

CURRENT CLINICAL PRACTICE

Neil S. Skolnik, MD, Series Editor

For other titles published in this series, go to
www.springer.com/series/7633

Pediatric Interviewing

A Practical, Relationship-Based Approach

James Binder, MD

Marshall University School of Medicine,
Huntington, WV, USA

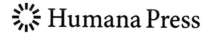 Humana Press

James Binder, MD
Marshall University School of Medicine
Huntington, WV
USA
binderj@marshall.edu

ISBN 978-1-60761-255-1   e-ISBN 978-1-60761-256-8
DOI 10.1007/978-1-60761-256-8
Springer New York Dordrecht Heidelberg London

Library of Congress Control Number: 2009944066

Printed on acid-free paper

Humana Press is part of Springer Science+Business Media (www.springer.com)

To
Susan, James, Michael, and Maura

In loving memory of Jim and
Pat Binder

Series Editor Introduction

Ὁβίος βραχύς, ἐ δε ἱἐχνη μακρή

Life is short, [the] art long
—Hippocrates

Pediatric Interviewing: A Practical, Relationship Based Approach by James Binder is filled with a unique blend of wisdom, experience, and evidence, which will serve as a guide and as a reminder that what comes first in the care of the patient is the language and the silences that are shared between patient and physician. The medical interview quickly establishes the type of caring relationship the two will share. In this age of electronic medical records, pay-forperformance, and evidence-based medicine it is easy to lose sight that medicine is fundamentally about one person who has knowledge and experience providing care for another individual who is asking for help. How the physician organizes his or her interactions has an important impact on the experience and outcomes for both the physician and for the patient.

Dr. Binder presents a conceptual framework with which to approach interviewing and illustrates this framework with practical examples from years of teaching and practice. Physicians-intraining will find this book filled with wisdom and much needed recommendations about how to approach the medical interview. For those of us who have been in practice a number of years, Dr. Binder's book can serve as a refreshing opportunity to reflect in detail about something many of us take for granted – the complexity of the medical interview. He reminds us that the medical interview has many goals in addition to the collection of information. These goals include establishing relationships with patients, educating patients, coming to an agreement with patients on therapeutic goals to enhance compliance, and leaving the door welcome and open for future follow-up.

This is an important book that comes at an important time. With all the current discussion about health care reform, it is refreshing to read a book about the most basic aspect of medicine, the medical interview, which can take a lifetime to perfect yet is practiced every day. Increasingly our method of recording information, in an electronic medical record, will force us to pay more and more attention to the *content* of the information we gather. This attention to content will make *Pediatric Interviewing* an ever more important book for physicians-in-training as well as those in practice, to help us keep our focus on the simple fact that the *process* of gathering information and forming relationships with our patients has inherent value. Done correctly, with empathy and attention to detail, this process makes both patient and physician feel more satisfied with the interaction and also affects health outcomes. The relationship that develops between a physician and a patient has a direct therapeutic effect, influences the information obtained, the decisions about what treatments a patient will consider, compliance with medications and lifestyle modification, and keeps the door open so that patients are comfortable returning for follow-up.

For a book so well written, so well thought-out, so insightful, and so timely, Dr. Binder deserves our thanks.

Neil S. Skolnik, MD

Foreword

It is well known to everyone who reads that our health care system in the USA is out of control. We spend almost two and half trillion (yes, that is with a "T") dollars on this system and yet 45 million Americans are uninsured. The system is inefficient, and medical errors occur much more commonly than we would like to believe. In no small measure, the exorbitant cost of health care contributes to our current economic crisis, the failing of small businesses, and lost wages of the American worker. And worst of all, despite all the amount of money spent on our health care system, by many measures, we are not healthier (and in many ways less healthy) than those in other industrialized countries.

So what in the world does this have to do with a book on pediatric interviewing? Well, the fact is that we are on the cusp of reevaluating how it is that we approach the delivery of health care. Health care reform has been and will continue to be a major debate over the next few years. This discussion will not just consider how to pay for our health care, but also how to structure the delivery of it. For years, we have shunned prevention and prided ourselves in our ever expanding technology and our ability to "fix" any disease that came along. That attitude is beginning to change as we recognize the costs involved. Promotion of healthy behaviors and prevention of disease must become a crucial part of our responsibilities as health care providers. And if we are going to be successful in this, we must start reemphasizing some basic tenets of medicine – most important of which is that good care begins with the establishment of a trusting doctor–patient relationship.

Somewhere between our increasing love affair with new technologies and creating health care provider networks ("you can see any of our 50 doctors – you just won't see the same one twice!") we have forgotten that good patient care is really about relationships. It is the relationship between a patient (or family) and a doctor that allows them to trust one another, feel for one another, and understand each other's stresses and problems. We teach young doctors how to talk TO their patients. But we do not really teach them how to talk WITH their patients. We may know what instructions to give, what topics to cover, and what check lists to complete when we see our patients. But how often are we really listening to them? How much time do we spend understanding why a patient does not follow our advice? Are we really having a two-way conversation when we provide this advice or are we preaching? I would submit that our ability to successfully create necessary behavior change in patients and families would be improved if we improve our communication skills. The net result of this will be more success in reducing the number of patients with preventable morbidities. And as an added bonus, better communication will also lead to increased job satisfaction by having patients who are thankful for our understanding and empathy.

This is why Jim's book should be essential reading – not only for all students but also for any physician working with children and families. It provides a wealth of practical tips for improving your interviewing skills. This includes all situations, from the simple provision of well-child care to difficult situations involving the hardest to reach patients.

I have always thought that it was strange that we talk about being "health care" providers. In fact, our training taught us very little about health and a lot about disease. And with the increasing strain on the doctor–patient relationship, it seems we are doing less and less "caring" than before. This is a book that brings us back to why most of us became doctors in the first place. It will teach you to communicate. It will teach you to understand. It will teach you to care.

Read it. Enjoy it. Learn from it.

Pittsburgh, PA   *Bob Cicco, MD*
                                              April, 2009

Preface

A good clinician needs to interview with efficiency and effectiveness. A clinician who cares for children must be able to join with families, understand their concerns, discern what is wrong with the sick child, and promote healthy development. An effective clinician who cares for children possesses and uses the skills needed for talking and listening to families. I intend this book for clinicians, young and old, who want to learn those skills. Since I work with trainees, I illustrate many teaching points in this text with examples from a training setting.

The evidence is extensive. Good communication has clear benefits for the clinician. Clinicians who interview well have a number of advantages, including the capability of gathering a full data base and of interviewing efficiently. These skills satisfy and fulfill clinicians, very important results [1]. Satisfied clinicians burn out less often and change careers less frequently. They are also more likely to be emotionally available and positively engaged with their patients. In turn, their patients report being satisfied with the clinicians and liking them more [2]. This leads them to file fewer lawsuits, a key benefit of relating well to patients, in view of the suffering clinician's experience when involved in a lawsuit [3]. Clinicians who interview well tend to enjoy medicine.

Satisfied patients are more likely to follow through with treatment plans and have improved health outcomes [3]. Barbara Korsch described this phenomenon over 30 years ago [2]. Interviewing effectiveness enhances physician–patient relationships, which in turn, impact health outcomes.

Child-oriented clinicians understand the importance of relationships. This importance surfaces as one of the key principles of developmental pediatrics. A child's first relationships with his caregivers form the secure base from which the child learns to explore, interact, and talk.

> Partnership is a reliable ally for the child in times of grief, anger, and frustration because it serves as a protection from despair and emotional collapse. ... Every aspect of the toddler's development

is influenced by the presence or absence of a secure base and a partnership between parent and child.

Alicia Lieberman [4]

The fact that a toddler handles adversity better when living in a healthy relationship should not surprise us. We might be surprised by the fact that sick patients do better when they benefit from a healthy partnership with their clinician. Research has demonstrated that patients with diabetes have lower glycosylated hemoglobins (HbA1c) and patients with hypertension have lower blood pressures when the patient/clinician partnership is healthy [3]. Exciting news! Relationships really do have the power to influence health. Thus, any theory of interviewing must be solidly based on relationship theory (see Appendix F).

This book begins with an analysis of the shut-down interview, one type of difficult medical interview. Such an analysis will help clarify the connection between relationship and communication. An interviewer has a number of ways to influence an interview in a positive direction, even a shut-down interview, if she maintains an empathic, respectful relationship with her patient.

References

1 Suchman AL, Roter D, Green M, Lipkin M, the Collaborative Study Group of the American Academy on Physician and Patient (1993) Physician satisfaction with primary care office visits. Med Care 31:1083–1092

2 Korsch BM, Aley EF (1973) Pediatric interviewing techniques: current pediatric therapy. Sci Am 3:1–42

3 Roter DL, Hall JA (2006) Doctors talking with patients/patients talking with doctors: improving communication in medical visits, 2nd edn. Praeger, Wesport, CT

4 Lieberman AF (1993) The emotional life of the toddler. Free Press, New York

Acknowledgments

I have been fortunate to learn from many gifted teachers. Vann Joines is a teaching supervisor of redecision therapy training at the Southeast Institute in Chapel Hill. He models compassion, humor, patience, and enjoyment of life. The principles of healthy relationships I learned in that setting shaped my understanding of relationships and interviewing. I modeled much of my teaching approach in Chap. 12 on what I experienced at the Southeast Institute over the last two decades.

Michael Rothenberg triggered my earliest interest in interviewing during a fellowship with him. A decade later, I became increasingly curious about interviewing after reading *Psychiatric Interviewing: The Art of Understanding* by Shawn Shea. I attended several workshops and seminars Shawn gave on interviewing and the teaching of interviewing. His influence is seen throughout the book.

I want to thank my editor, Richard Lansing, who had confidence in my manuscript even before I did and nurtured me along the entire process.

Jody Sondheimer, Barbara Korsch, Diana Peticca, Tim Murphy, Doris Murphy, and Joseph Werthammer read the entire manuscript. I appreciate their time, expertise, and valuable suggestions.

Many readers read sections of the book. Again, they were generous with their encouragement and helpful recommendations. These included Linda Cooper, Elmer Holzinger, Tom Ellis, Ina Binder, Jenna Dolan, Bob Miller, Ed Pino, Joseph Evans, Holly Cloonan, Charlotte Jones, Mark Wippel, and Debbie Lilly.

Ada Olah and Barbara Dalton provided expert technical assistance with patience and good humor. The Marshall University Department of Pediatrics provided strong support for my project.

I am indebted to my patients and families for sharing their stories with me. The stories in the book may reflect lessons I have learned from the families I have been honored to meet. They do not reflect any particular patient or family.

I received unwavering encouragement from my spouse, Susan, our three children, James, Michael, and Maura, as well as our entire extended family. I started the book at the suggestion of Michael. James offered much needed technical help. I am particularly grateful to Susan, who read the manuscript too many times to count, patiently listened to me, edited, consulted, and loved me throughout the 3-year project. Anyone who has lived with a spouse writing a book knows that is no easy task.

A SPECIAL THANKS

I feel a sense of pleasure saying thanks to Fred Platt. Fred responded to an e-mail request from a stranger (me) with an inspiring openness. He mentored me with generosity, wisdom, and patience. I was lucky to receive the benefit of his knowledge of medicine and patient–physician relationships. In addition, Fred taught me many skills essential for writing a book. I am deeply grateful. He and his warm, delightful wife, Connie, even opened up their home to Susan and me for a weekend of editing and fun.

Fred's influence is so strong throughout the book that anytime I use the word "we" I really am referring to Fred and myself.

Contents

I
The Shut-Down Interview and Relationships

I think people respond to joy and work and love and achievement and learning and appreciation and gratitude–and a sense of a job well done. I think that it feels good to be a good doctor and better to be a better doctor.

Don Berwick

Case: Amy is a second year pediatric resident who just had a difficult night covering the NICU. She has continuity clinic this morning and expects a full schedule of patients. Her first patient is Henry, a 9-year-old, slightly pudgy boy with a history of encoporesis. Henry makes no eye contact with Amy. Amy tries to appear friendly and attempts to *join* with Henry. Henry grunts several one word responses, never looking at Amy. Amy quickly recognizes a shut-down interview in this opening phase. Fortunately, Amy is curious. What is going on with Henry?

1. Does he just have a shy, anxious type of personality?
2. Is he depressed?
3. Does he dislike me?
4. Did his custodial aunt force him to come for the checkup and he feels upset and angry?
5. Is he quiet because he is experiencing shame related to his encoporesis?
6. Is there another explanation I have not thought of?

Amy bases these possible explanations for the shut-down interview by imagining what Henry could be feeling or experiencing

J. Binder, *Pediatric Interviewing: A Practical, Relationship-Based Approach*, Current Clinical Practice, DOI 10.1007/978-1-60761-256-8_1,
© Springer Science+Business Media, LLC 2010

underneath his withdrawn behavior. Any theory of a shut-down interview must take the underlying feelings of the patient into account. Since those underlying feelings are seldom clearly apparent, the clinician must use her imagination and then check back with the patient to validate her ideas.

The clinician who has a clear concept of the dynamics of a shut-down interview has a number of options for opening up the patient. Fundamentally, a patient withdraws or shuts down from others, rather than express his feelings, when he does not feel emotionally safe expressing those feelings. Likely, he learned this way of relating in his family-of-origin. The clinician cannot change the patient's childhood experience. However, she can provide emotional safety in the present.

Children of any age may shut down. The young frightened child, the shy preadolescent, and the coerced adolescent, harboring anger and resentment, present common scenarios in any pediatric practice. Parents, too, may shut down.

Since each patient has his or her own unique reasons for not opening up to the examiner, the management of each situation must be individualized. What works in one situation may not work in another. A consecutive string of 5–6 open-ended questions often opens up adult patients [1]. A consecutive string of open-ended questions can feel invasive and probing to a fiercely independent adolescent and be ineffective [1]. In a similar fashion, long pauses typically are ineffective with rebellious teenagers, while long pauses might result in activation of an adult [1].

A shut-down interview directly and totally blocks two core tasks of a medical interview.

- Engaging the patient
- Activating the patient to provide an accurate and thorough history

RECOGNITION OF THE SHUT-DOWN INTERVIEW
If the interviewer stays aware of the process as well as the content, she usually will recognize the existence of a shut-down interview; in fact, she will find it painfully obvious. Many types of body responses signal blocked communication and can be clues to a possible shut-down interview. For example, a shut-down patient might display infrequent or nonexistent eye contact, immobile or tight facial muscles, a closed body posture – folded arms, crossed legs, wearing a coat indoors – or body positioning turned away from the physician [1]. The patient's verbal responses then confirm the presence (or absence) of a shut-down interview. Verbal clues

to a shut-down interview include little or no elaboration when an open-ended question is asked, delayed responses, short and snappy answers, and no spontaneous conversation [1].

MANAGEMENT OF THE SHUT-DOWN INTERVIEW
Recognizing a shut-down interview during the opening phase allows the physician to deal with the process. The clinician needs to change the process *before* moving on to other tasks. The completeness and accuracy of the data collection depend on resolving this issue [1]. One must first establish emotional safety in the opening phase of the interview, an especially important task in a shut-down interview. We support emotional safety by:

1. Staying aware of our own emotions and maintaining a nonjudgmental stance.
2. Tracking with the patient
3. Establishing a clear contract (agenda) for the session
4. Acknowledging and validating the patient's feelings
5. Affirming the patient's movement in a positive direction [2]

Each of these actions offers the clinician an option for interviewing with a shut-down patient.

1. Amy, the exhausted second year resident, highlights the importance of staying self-aware, not getting distracted with thoughts about past or future events, so that she is free to follow the patient's lead (tracking). Mindful that she was physically and emotionally spent after a night on call in the Newborn Intensive fCare Unit (NICU), Amy knew that she faced a challenge with her continuity clinic patients. Amy had a plan. She had learned during her busy first year of residency that by slowing down a bit, taking a few slow breaths, she could recognize what she was thinking and feeling in the present moment and then manage those feelings.

   Amy is aware that she is feeling mildly annoyed as she looks at her list of continuity patients. She is imagining that Henry is still be symptomatic, maybe because his aunt is not following through with the treatment plan. The aunt has been inconsistent in the past. Amy manages her annoyance by reminding herself that her aunt is likely doing the best that she can. And, it is not her job to judge the aunt anyway. Amy realizes that it will be challenging for her to maintain a nonjudgmental stance when she is so tired.

   Amy does all this before she enters the room to see Henry and his aunt. She is calm and focused. Since shut-down interviews have such a powerful ability to trigger anxiety and discomfort in the interviewer, this is a significant accomplishment. Patients readily sense physician's frustration. Typically, their withdrawal then becomes more deeply entrenched. Roter and Hall describe a negative spiral effect of patients not feeling accepted (or liked) by their physicians. They note poor outcomes, both poorer communication between physicians and patients, and poor health outcomes for patients [3].

Amy notices Henry's nonverbal communication. He is sitting in a slouched position, head downcast and not making eye contact. She intuits that Henry is experiencing one of the feelings – shame – that she had considered as a possible stimulus for the shut-down interview. She will check out that intuition later in the interview by using a normalization technique. For now, Amy helps establish a safe atmosphere by taking a nonjudgmental, accepting stance.

2. Establishing a clear *contract* for working together supports a true partnership between a physician and patient. We may skip right past the contract as a natural response to the uneasiness typically felt during a shut-down interview. But, the interviewer cannot really move to the next step without addressing this issue. Several possibilities exist:

- Make the withdrawn behavior overt and label it as okay. The patient is given permission not to talk [4]. That is the contract.

  "Its okay if you don't talk. I'll talk to mom. If you change your mind and want to join in, please feel free to do so."

  This approach can increase cooperation in a variety of settings – a fearful young child, a rebellious teenager – essentially, the patient is given time to feel comfortable and make a choice whether to participate in the interview.

- As a corollary of the above approach, the clinician can piggyback a question about her wishes. Again, their withdrawn behavior is labeled in an okay manner.

  "I understand you do not want to be here. Given that you do not want to be here, is there anything that you want to ask or have checked today?"

  Thus, a direct request for the patient's input – a prerequisite for a valid contract.

- As a third contracting option, the interviewer can state what she herself wants out of the visit [4].

"I am interested in everybody's opinion. It will help me understand better if you tell me your view of the problem."

- Before leaving the area of contracting, Bonnie Ramsey offers yet another option when dealing with a resistant teenager saying "I don't know" to all inquiries. To paraphrase Dr. Ramsey:

  I'd like to make a deal with you. I'll be straight with you and you be straight with me. I know you are too smart to not know the answer to questions I ask. So instead of saying "I don't know" like a lot of adolescents I see, would you agree to say "I won't answer that" if you don't want to respond? [5]

  The adolescent patient may decide that he is willing to answer questions when asked in an open straight forward way. Even if he decides not to answer, communication has been open and honest – a prerequisite for a valid contract.

- Finally according to Vann Joines (May 2005) a resistant teenager saying "I don't know" will sometimes respond to the playful response of the interviewer.

  "If you did know…"

3. An *empathic* stance provides another whole category of responses to a shut-down interview. It is difficult to elicit and acknowledge a patient's experience and feelings when he is not talking. One needs a little creativity and cleverness. A clinician might use the third person technique to get at the patient's feelings underneath the defensive, withdrawn position [6].

   "Henry, lots of children don't want to talk to the doctor when they didn't want to come in the first place. They say to themselves, 'You can make me come, but you can't make me talk.' Is that true for you?"
   "Lots of times when parents expected to see their regular pediatrician and find they unexpectedly have been assigned to a different pediatrician in the group, they feel disappointed or even annoyed. Is that true for you?"

   As another option, the clinician can respond empathically to the patient's nonverbal communication of his feelings. For example, the rebelliousness of a child or teenager, who did not want to come to the doctor and would not talk, can be acknowledged and validated.

> "Henry, I can see nothing I say is going to get you to talk. You're really good at not talking."

It is important that this is expressed with a sincere appreciation of Henry's rebelliousness and not conveyed as frustration with Henry.

4. Finally, we can affirm a shut-down patient, our last category of responses. On first glance, it might appear that affirming a silent patient would be difficult, if not impossible. Not true! We just saw an example of a physician smoothly affirming and acknowledging Henry's experience.

In *Transforming the Difficult Child*, Howard Glasser describes a technique for affirming children who are difficult to reach with typical approaches. He coined the term "video moment" for his technique [7]. A parent uses neutral language to describe in detail the everyday activities of a child. The power of the technique is a result of the parent *noticing* the child. The fact that the parent makes a neutral statement – not critical or praising – allows it to be taken in by children who reject both criticism and praise. The detail of the parent's remark convinces the child that the parent is noticing them – when things are not going wrong. Glasser calls this technique "The Nurtured Heart Approach" since the everyday goodness of the child is being affirmed. A physician can use this same method of affirming a young child.

> "Henry, I noticed you walked right into the room and climbed upon the exam table. You're sitting quietly and looking at me. You seem to be listening to what I am saying."

A second method of affirming a shut-down patient is to talk about *any* subject for which the patient expresses an interest – music, soccer, items in the exam room. A child who is reluctant to talk is more likely to open up on a concrete, familiar topic than his or her feelings [4]. Children feel cared for and affirmed when adults are genuinely interested in what they are doing and saying.

PITFALLS

Attempting to force a patient to talk would not be an appropriate response based on the ethical principle of autonomy. However, physicians stressed by lack of time or other constraints easily fall into this trap. Trying to force a patient to talk will not work, of course. Leaning on someone leads to resistance.

I believe the flip side of forcing the issue – doing nothing at all – is an equally unnecessary pitfall. Giving up and thinking

"What's the use?" leads to the same results as forcing the issue. In my time supervising residents and students, I have seen this interview response frequently. If a resident believes she has no power to influence the course of the interview, then she will not change the interview process. And, we have just seen that a shut-down interview is not a hopeless situation. The interviewer has options that work reasonably well.

Amy's transactions with Henry and his family help demonstrate the key principles that I accept as *core assumptions* in this text:

1. Communication is the external manifestation of what is being experienced in that relationship. In addition, communication creates that relationship in the first place.
2. Medical interviewing has unique features that make it different from other forms of interviewing.
3. The family is the patient.
4. A reciprocal connection between the physical and mental exists. Therefore, we should approach health care from a biopsychosocial perspective to understand the patient's experience of illness and health.
5. We can teach and we can learn the complex skill we call *The Medical Interview*.

References

1. Shea SC (1998) Psychiatric interviewing: the art of understanding: a practical guide for psychiatrists, psychologists, nurses and other health professionals, 2nd edn. WB Saunders, Philadelphia
2. Joines V (1997) Accessing the natural child as the key to redecision therapy. In: Lennox C (ed) Redecision therapy: a brief, action-oriented approach. Jason Aronson, Northvale, NJ
3. Roter DL, Hall JA (2006) Doctors talking with patients/patients talking with doctors: improving communication in medical visits, 2nd edn. Praeger, Westport, CT
4. Anderson CM, Stewart S (1983) Mastering resistance: a practical guide to family therapy. Guilford, New York
5. Interviewing tip of the month. Training Institute for Suicide Assessment and Clinical Interviewing. No. 60, February 2005. http://www.testflight.net/suicideassessment/catalog/archives.php. Accessed 8 Oct 2007
6. Kohlberg I, Rothenberg MB (1970) Comprehensive care following multiple life-threatening injuries. Am J Dis Child 119:449–451
7. Glasser H, Easley J (1998) Transforming the difficult child: the nurtured heart approach. Vaughan, Nashville, TN

2

The Medical Interview: The Opening Phase

Organizing is what you do before you do something, so that when you do it, it is not all mixed up.

A.A. Milne

Case: Becky is a 9-year-old girl who presents to the clinic with mid-thoracic back pain of 3-weeks duration. She arrives accompanied by her 36-year-old single, divorced mother, Mrs. Torri. Mrs. Torri and Becky sit next to each other on the same chair even though an empty chair is nearby. Mrs. Torri spontaneously starts talking after the clinician introduces himself. She is somewhat hurried as she skips from topic to topic – from the back pain to Becky's posture to her ex-husband.

The clinician, Tom, a first year pediatric resident, must make a decision only one minute into the interview. Does he track with Mrs. Torri as she goes from topic to topic? This may lead to inadequate data regarding the back pain. Should he focus on the back pain risking decreasing rapport with the mother? And, maybe the psychosocial data has a role to play in the etiology of the back pain. Tom needs a structure which will allow him to develop and maintain a strong engagement, efficiently obtain the specific characteristics of the back pain in order to make an accurate diagnosis, and discuss the diagnosis and possible treatment with the family.

Fred Platt notes that one should take a deep breath before trying to describe anything as complex as a clinical interview. It is surely not an easy task. Part of the problem stems from the multidimensional nature of a clinical interview. Per conversation with Platt, it is

J. Binder, *Pediatric Interviewing: A Practical, Relationship-Based Approach,* Current Clinical Practice, DOI 10.1007/978-1-60761-256-8_2, © Springer Science+Business Media, LLC 2010

useful to consider three dimensions*: the tools used by the clinician, the goals of the interview, and the topics to be considered in the conversation (March 2009). Closely allied to the topics considered are the data we seek to understand.

1. *The tools used* by a clinician include many that are seldom described in interview manuals and may be seldom appreciated. They range from allowing the patient the freedom to tell whatever he wishes to an entirely controlled question-and-answer format. Clinicians do many things in conversing with a patient. They may listen, invite stories, give orders, use gentle commands, urge, disregard, echo, summarize, empathize, facilitate, ask closed or open questions, use focused or wide-ranging questions and directions, or even argue with or disregard their patients. Of course, some of these techniques are likely to please the patient (e.g. sustained listening) and some likely to displease (e.g. arguing and disregarding); some are likely to uncover hidden facts (e.g. closed questions) and some more likely to lead to an understanding of the patient's personality, his values, feelings, and ideas (e.g. gentle commands or invitations to talk).

2. *The functions of the interview* do include data retrieval. But they also include building rapport, a working relationship with the patient. And they include forward future moves such as educating the patient, reaching a plan with the patient, and enlisting the patient in his own health measures for the future [1]. Some of our techniques tend to build rapport. These include understanding the patient's emotional issues and empathizing with them, seeking to know the patient's values, and listening intently and for enough time to lead the patient to feel heard. Some of our techniques seem to damage rapport and lead to less patient cooperation in the future. Such behaviors, unfortunately used all too often, include rushing the patient through the story, disregarding what has been said, arguing and bullying tactics.

3. *The data desired* by the clinician may include the patient's personal story, the cardinal symptom (chief complaint), symptom descriptors, including associated symptoms, other active health concerns and symptoms, past medical events, family history, health hazards and healthy behaviors, existence of family discord or violence, religious or other transcendental concerns, nutritional practices, and so on (Platt).

A popular approach to structuring is to differentiate *patient-centered* interviewing from *doctor-centered*, a model that tends to combine the data desired with the tools used [2]. In such a model the personal story of the patient may be inquired about using open-ended inquiry, but the further medical data are largely obtained by closed questioning. Despite the helpfulness of this model, we do not believe it is adequate to explain the much more complex sequence that clinicians use. In this chapter, we will talk about the first of the three phases of the interview, the opening or patient-centered phase, sometimes focusing on one dimension of the medical interview in order to clarify a technique, a skill, and a goal or task. We stress the need to view the medical interview in the three dimensions described above as we follow the procedures and techniques we might use in such a conversation during the opening and subsequent phases.

We might consider particles from clinical interviews:

Dr: Can you tell me the story of the illness?

Parent: Sure! He started coughing three nights ago and the cough is getting more bothersome. It's loud and he just coughs on and on. Nothing comes up and he has no fever but I'm worried about him.

[In this morsel from a clinical interview the clinician uses an *invitation to tell the story* as a technique, is likely to increase rapport by that open-ended query, and focuses on the data (symptoms) of the present illness.]
Or

Dr: It sounds as if his cough is really worrying you. What sort of concerns does it bring up for you?

Parent: Well, I've heard that whooping cough is going around again. And you're right. I am scared.

[In this piece of interview, the clinician uses an empathic summary and an open-ended inquiry about the parent's own diagnosis for the child. Again likely to increase trust and rapport but focusing on feelings and ideas rather than symptoms.]
Or

Dr: Does he have chest pain? Trouble breathing? Fever?

Parent: No, no fever.

[This clinician uses closed-ended questions, seeking some specific data about symptoms, a technique that may lead to only the last question being answered and an ambivalent parent, one who may value the clinician's thoroughness and at the same time one who may feel oppressed by the technique (Platt)].

Given these three dimensions, we consider the **tasks of the opening phase**.

1. Creating a working relationship with the family and the patient, one based on mutual respect and trust
2. Establishing emotional safety
3. Checking own internal emotional experience
4. Activating the family to give their perception of the problem
5. Evaluating the *process* of the interview, itself [3]
6. Obtaining the family's full agenda, organizing and prioritizing it, and explaining your plan for the rest of the interview to the family

INTRODUCTION

The chief purpose of the introductory phase of the interview is straightforward: establish contact with the family. A friendly greeting helps put the family at ease [4]. Korsch documented many instances of physicians not even introducing themselves in her pioneering research on pediatric interviewing. A typical opening remark was:

"What seems to be the trouble?" [4]

This led to a focus on disease, not the person. The first issue in any interview is *contact*. Contact can be blocked by either the interviewer or the patient. A clinician might be worried about a personal problem or occupied with another clinical situation, such as a child on the inpatient ward. The clinician must recognize this and get himself fully present to enter the exam room and introduce himself. Conversely, a patient/family might not be fully present and ready to start the encounter. Perhaps, a parent is on a cell phone or distracted by young, active siblings. Whatever the situation, it must be resolved so that contact can be established. Contact is a Gestalt therapy term referring to the extent to which a person is aware and attuned to his own internal experience and how open he is to **listen** to the experience of others. Platt and Gordon note that:

"Many of us spend the time when another person is talking planning for what we will say next. That is not listening" [5].

In this interviewing text, we use the word contact simply to refer to the process of being **emotionally** connected to the experience of the other person.

Computers in the exam room are the most recent block to emotional contact. But before computers, we were burdened by our hand-written charts or our dictation of notes. Either could diminish the connection between clinician and patient/family.

OPENING
The opening steps include hearing the patient's personal story and the initial symptom data *and* setting the agenda. The opening fills that part of the interview between the introduction and the exploration of a specific topic or topics by the clinician with detailed questions about data not mentioned by the patient [3]. The clinician does not talk a lot during the opening phase. However, he is active mentally: listening, observing, assessing, and facilitating [3]. This phase of the interview may be brief or extended; perhaps, an average time to complete this phase would be from 3 to 5 mins. The clinician asks for the patient's chief complaint and any other concerns, elicits the personal context of the symptoms within the family, and develops an emotional focus. Smith emphasizes that this biopsychosocial approach is evidence-based and is more likely to result in full data collection than would a simply biological approach [2].

The clinician asks the patient/family for any other concerns more than once so that all problems are identified early and the agenda for the interview prioritized [2]. During this time the clinician learns why the family came at this time and a rough outline of the time frame of the symptoms. As the clinician obtains the list of problems, he often will find it helpful to limit the patient's desire to talk about details of a symptom until the entire agenda is known [2].

> "The headaches are important. We will come back to them, but I first want to see if you have any other concerns"

Once the clinician has a list of all the concerns or problems that need to be dealt with during the visit, he develops the **personal context** of the symptoms [2]. He learns about the *illness,* not just the underlying disease. The personal context of the illness includes the day-to-day family context, such as school or activity plans, as well as stresses such as grief, loss, and family or job problems [2]. The clinician invites the family to tell their personal story with an open-ended question like:

> "Given what you have told me, how are you doing?" [2]

Often, a family will give the clinician personal information in small chunks. The clinician repeatedly focuses on these pieces of information in order to elicit the full story [2]. It is important to avoid focusing too prematurely on further defining the physical symptoms at this stage [2]. We return to our case example from the introduction to the chapter.

Case: Becky is that 9-year-old girl with mid-thoracic back pain we met at the beginning of the chapter. We join the interview after their agreement on the contract for the clinic visit.

Physician: So, what has it been like for you Mrs. Torri with Becky having back pain over the last month?

Mrs. Torri: Well, the pain doesn't go away.

Comment: The physician *avoids* asking her to further characterize the symptom at this point. If the patient does further characterize the symptom the physician listens and moves to the personal context when the opportunity arises. Mrs. Torri seems worried about the cause of the pain, so the physician asks her about that.

Physician: What are you most concerned about?

Mrs. Torri: I wonder why she still has the pain.

Physician: And, what concerns you about it lasting this long?

Mrs. Torri: Maybe it's serious, something wrong with her spine.

Physician: So, if I understand you right, you're picturing all sorts of terrible problems involving her spine. I see. You worry about Becky. I promise that we will return to your concern after I finish my exam.

Mrs. Torri: Okay

Physician: You have been concerned. What else has it been like
for you?

Comment: The physician addressed the worry, then persisted in obtaining further personal data.

Mrs. Torri: Well, I keep telling her to watch her posture. She's always leaning over to draw pictures.

Physician: Becky, you like to draw?

Comment: The physician uses *echoing* to invite Becky to expand on this tidbit of personal data

Becky: I love to draw.

Mrs. Torri: She's very good.

Physician: Becky, how did you get interested in drawing?

Becky: I don't know. My mom draws, too.

Mrs. Torri:	I do love to draw also. The difference is Becky won't do anything else. She has poor posture from drawing so much and she won't go out and play.
Physician:	Tell me more. (*gentle command*)
Mrs. Torri:	She doesn't get enough exercise. She will go out to play and be back in the house in five minutes.
Physician:	Becky, what do you think about what mom is saying?
Becky:	It's true.
Physician:	Mrs. Torri, it sounds like you and Becky share a love of drawing. I can imagine that is a great joy to both of you. You think she is a good artist, but is drawing too much. You believe this is leading to poor posture and possibly back pain, as well as a lack of exercise (*summarization*).
Mrs. Torri:	That's right. I don't know how to get her to play more.
Physician:	What have you tried?
Mrs. Torri:	I tell her to go play.
Physician:	What happens?
Mrs. Torri:	She only plays for a few minutes.
Physician:	What do you think the reason for this is?
Mrs. Torri:	I don't think she likes to play by herself. Plus, she worries about me.
Physician:	She worries about you. (**echoing**)
Mrs. Torri:	She always is worried about me. She worries because I smoke and have had medical problems.
Comment:	The physician has deepened the personal story using echoing, gentle commands, and summarization (we will discuss these techniques shortly) – whenever the family mentioned any personal information. It took only a few minutes. These techniques invite the family to expand the story in whatever direction they choose [2]. The physician does not introduce new material during the open phase of the interview. In this instance, the physician not only enhanced his relationship with this family, but also he learned information about what might be producing the symptom.

Sometimes, a family is slow to reveal their personal story. Novice interviewers frequently react to this *block* by avoiding the patient's personal story and moving directly to defining the physical symptoms. Often these interviewers hold onto a belief that they are being intrusive (or unpleasant) by asking for the personal story, might lose control of the interview, or that the family will bring up emotional issues they will not be able to handle [2]. Yet, a student must persist and resolve whatever block exists. The ability of a clinician to obtain a full data base depends on his relationship with the patient [2]. A relationship can only evolve by getting to know the patient/family. That means eliciting the personal story. Families welcome a personal connection with their clinicians [6]. Clinicians who learn the personal context of a patient's story do not lose control.

If a family does not respond to the techniques used in the above example (echoing, gentle commands, summarization), the interviewer has other options. One very effective option is to *simply to tell the family what is needed*:

> "I like to get to know families personally before discussing the physical symptoms. I find it helpful to place the symptoms within a personal context. I will gather specific information about the symptoms in a few minutes. Is that okay?"

We use this option frequently, and I have never encountered a family that did not agree to this request. Of course, when a child needs immediate attention (e.g., respiratory distress), the clinician postpones the personal context. *In situations in which the patient expects to give biomedical data immediately, such as in the emergency room, the personal data can be elicited at a later point in the visit*. As the clinician gathers the personal story, he is in a good position to elicit and empathize with the patient's emotional response. Empathy solidifies engagement with the patient, one of the six major tasks or goals of the opening phase of the interview.

EMOTIONAL SAFETY/ENGAGEMENT

As the clinician listens to the patient's and parent's perspective, he simultaneously works to establish emotional safety. We create a sense of safety when the patient or parent feels accepted and not judged. Feeling safe helps a patient become engaged and talk. In fact, if the patient is not personally engaged and given space to talk, there is a real risk that the data base will be incomplete [7]. This can take time, especially if the patient has had previous medical or life experiences of not being accepted. Strategies that have been shown to enhance safety include the following:

- Establishing a clear *contract*
- Listening/tracking with the patient
- Conveying empathetic understanding
  Making positive statements regarding what they are doing well [8]

A **contract** is an agreement between two or more people to a course of action. Each person knows what is expected of them [9]. No surprises! Encounters in which personal, intimate information is being shared, as are most medical interactions, require such a contract.

Case: A 9-month-old baby is in the clinic for a failure-to-thrive assessment. The clinician knows that he must gather both physical and psychosocial data to evaluate this baby. He will need information about family relationships.

Clinician: I hear you are concerned about your baby not gaining weight over the last three months. I imagine this must be difficult for you. Babies not gaining weight can be caused by a number of different conditions, from chronic infections to gastrointestinal problems. We also know that stresses families face can be important in how a baby is growing. So, I will be asking you a number of questions about Sarah's health, as well as questions about how things are going for you as a family. Is that okay?

Parents: Yes.

This way the parents will not be surprised by questions about family relationships. They will be more likely to collaborate with the clinician in his effort to find the source of the problem. Sometimes, a contract is implicit. For example, a child comes to the doctor with fever and lethargy. The implicit contract is that the doctor will do a competent history and physical exam and accurately diagnose the child. Even this type of contract can be made overt, so there are no surprises.

"So you are concerned about Emily's fever. Is there anything else that you wanted us to address during this visit? Were there any specific sorts of conditions that you were particularly concerned about?"

Part of the contract needs to address the time available for the visit so that both parties can plan accordingly [2]. Then we must discuss the issue of *confidentiality* with an adolescent and her family as still another aspect of contracting:

"What we talk about, Tom, is between you and me. I will not tell your parents what you say unless I become concerned over your safety or the safety of someone else. In that case, I would talk to you about it first. Do we have an agreement?"

TRACKING

Tracking refers to the process of commenting on, or asking a question, about the patient's immediately preceding statement. It *ties* the patient's world, including his way of understanding his problems, to our need to obtain the medical data needed for diagnosis [10]. Sometimes the tie is a summarization of what the patient has so far told you. It can also be a short utterance like "I see," "So, you are..." giving the patient that evidence that the clinician is listening to what he just said and believes it is important.

Mother: My baby doesn't latch on to the breast very well. I'm worried she is not getting enough milk.

Clinician: I see. Tell me more about that.

Occasionally, a patient may express something remarkable (e.g. "My husband walked out the door yesterday."). A response like "Oh my" lets the patient know the clinician is a caring human being and is listening [5].

Tracking a patient's statements and feelings is a fundamental counseling principle. It allows the interviewer to understand the patient's emotional experience, *a prerequisite understanding for expressing empathy*, the most powerful tool the clinician has for enhancing engagement. But, what should the clinician do if the patient does not express emotion during this early part of the interview? Smith recommends adopting *emotion-seeking skills* because of the importance of solidly engaging with the patient [2]. A clinician using a *direct* emotion-seeking skill might simply ask the patient:

"What has that been like for you?"

Recently, a resident and I saw a family to evaluate their child for failure to thrive. The mother responded immediately to the above inquiry with tears and an expression of her deep fear about what this means for her baby. Prior to that question, she appeared guarded. Afterward, she became fully engaged with us. Asking about underlying worries or concerns is another and important example of a direct inquiry into emotional content:

"What are you most worried about?"
"Why does that worry you?" [4]

Many parents bringing ill children to the doctor are worried about a serious underlying problem.

Indirect ways of eliciting the patient's emotional response can be useful with guarded patients. A patient can be asked what effect the condition has had on the patient or his family [2]. Often a family accesses vulnerable feelings as they report the impact of the condition on their child or family A very useful technique for eliciting feelings, which combines features of both indirect and direct approaches, is the *third-person technique*. The interviewer intuits that a patient is experiencing a certain feeling. He then says

"Lot's of children feel scared when they come to the doctor's.
Is that true for you?"

Many patients will be willing to share their experience once it has been normalized [11].

EMPATHY

Empathy has such an incredible power to increase contact and solidify engagement that Shea suggests making at least one empathic statement (*after* eliciting the feeling) in the first 5 mins [3]. Empathic understanding is the act of entering a patient's emotional experience while maintaining an objective perspective – "one foot in and one foot out." It is conveyed through nonverbal behavior and verbal statements that acknowledge, reflect, or normalize a patient's feelings and experience. Nonverbal expression of empathy may be the most important [1]. Since empathy is a response to the patient's immediate feeling, its power stems from responding to the patient's emotional experience *in the moment*. Anytime that a patient spontaneously expresses emotion, the clinician responds.

Cole and Bird recommend the use of two basic types of empathetic statements to clinicians: reflection and normalization.

Reflection is simply accurately acknowledging the words and emotional experience of another [1].

"It sounds like you have really worried about Joey."

or

"If I am hearing you right, you are annoyed with Jeremy's teacher"

or

"It looks like this is upsetting to you."

or

"You look sad."

Normalization lets the patient know that his feelings are understandable [1].

"No wonder you have been frustrated."

or

"Anyone would be angry in this situation."

or

"Of course you have grief. It's a big loss."

Or

"I can imagine how that would feel."

These methods of expressing empathy are not likely to threaten the patient by implying levels of emotion greater than the patient is willing to acknowledge [1].

Platt and Platt emphasize the importance of giving clear evidence to the patient that his ideas, values, and feelings/experience have been fully heard and understood. They recommend 5–10 s of **silence** after an empathic statement to allow the patient time to absorb the impact of the words. The final piece of the empathy cycle is asking and obtaining confirmation from the patient that the clinician has understood accurately [12].

AFFIRMATIONS

Closely related to empathetic statements are *affirmations* given to the patient. Affirmations flow from the philosophical conviction that all people have an okay essence or core. Affirmations must be *taken in* by the patient to be effective. They must fit in with the frame of reference of the patient or they will be rejected [9]. For example, a patient who believes she is an inadequate mother will likely reject a general statement such as:

"You're a wonderful mother."

She will have a much harder time rejecting a positive statement based on a specific behavior she is demonstrating right in the present moment [13].

"You hold the baby securely. He is feeling nurtured by you."

or

"I see you enjoy reading to Mary. That's a wonderful way for her to learn the love of books."

Affirmations, like empathy, are powerful ways to enhance engagement, a crucial task of the opening phase. They can be given for positive motivation even when a child or parent exhibits ineffective behaviors. For example, a parent who acknowledges that she is anxious and tends to hover and not support her child's independence can be told:

> "You are devoted to your child. It is clear that you care very much and want the best for her."

ACTIVATE FAMILIES TO GIVE THEIR PERCEPTION OF THE PROBLEM

The behavior of the clinician has a powerful influence on a patient's willingness to become **active** and give his perception of the problem. Communication researchers find two areas of nonverbal behavior of particular interest: proxemics and paralanguage.

Proxemics has to do with the effect of space and objects in a room on how participants relate. Edward Hall described a connection between the physical distance between people and their comfort level [14]. Shawn Shea discovered that 90% of the time interviewers felt most comfortable when seated 4–5 ft apart with the chairs turned 5–10° from a direct line between them. In other words, they did not face each directly in a confrontational manner, but seemed to be facing in the same direction in a collaborative way [3]. Astute clinicians make use of this information to set up the area they will be using for interviewing – a clinic exam room, an office, or even an inpatient room.

Paralanguage has to do with how something is said. For instance, consider a busy pediatrician who taps his fingers and rushes his questions. The patient might interpret the nonverbal communication to mean:

> "Don't ask any questions. I'm too busy to listen"

As a result, the patient does not respond to the pediatrician's verbalization

> "Do you have any questions?"

Whenever a mismatch exists between the verbal and nonverbal messages, people typically respond to the nonverbal message [15]. Every medical student is taught to adopt an even pace and calm tone of voice. Patients often respond to a calm, slow pace with a willingness to talk [3]. They respond less well to a clinician who hurries his patients, a behavior that may stem from any of the following: messages to *hurry* that physician received in his own childhood, modeling experienced during training when harried residents and faculty rush patients, or an overwhelming sense of *not enough time* that leads to the haste that makes waste, and in the process alienates and silences patients. These are powerful influences. It takes sustained effort by any clinician wanting to change that pattern. Such a clinician must stay aware of his own pace and make changes when needed.

VERBALIZATIONS

The words of the clinician make a difference too. Some types of verbalizations, such as facilitations and summarization, tend to activate patients. Head nodding, saying "uh-huh" or "I see" and echoing back the exact words of the patient ("Your baby won't stop crying") are examples of facilitations. Facilitations include verbal and non-verbal components [2]. Summarizing what the family has so far told the clinician encourages them to say more [2]. Facilitations and summarizing invite the family to talk without narrowing the focus. In fact, we can define *open-ended inquiry* as a process that helps the patient tell his story and then lets him know what we have heard and understood. Some writers describe open-ended inquiry as a combination of inviting the patient to tell a story, careful attentive listening, and then summarization of what is heard, all this followed again by more invitations, more listening, and more summaries [5]. "Let me see if I have heard you right. Sarah has had cough, headache, and fever for one day. She seems real tired. You are worried that she has the flu and that this will lead to breathing problems and a bad asthma attack, like she used to experience when she was younger. Is that right?" The clinician then pauses for 5-10 seconds to let the empathetic summary have an impact on the mother and give her a chance to say more. It is helpful to distinguish questions that are truly open from questions that, at first glance, appear open but are not. Two types of questions/statements are open-ended:

- Questions that begin with what or how, and by not asking for a specific answer, cannot be answered in one or two words [3].

  "How will you deal with this pressure from your friends?"
  "What kind of activities do you do for fun?"

  Yet we can note that:

  "What medication are you taking?"

  is an example of a closed-ended question. The answer set (medications) is limited.

- Gentle commands. They begin with "Tell me..." or "Describe...", and use a gentle, curious tone of voice [3].

"Tell me what you plan to do about the situation."

"Describe your relationship with your father."

Note: Gentle commands are powerful. This technique may be the single best tool a clinician can use to encourage a patient to divulge important matters [3].

Shea points out that several question types that seem open are not. Among his examples:

Swing questions– Answering the question can lead to a brief response as easily as activation of the patient. A swing question takes the form:

"Can you tell me...?"

Of course, in ordinary discourse a question like "Can you tell me how to get to the airport?" would not be answered with a "yes" or "no." A reasonable person would take it as a gentle request for a set of directions or a map. Similarly, a well-engaged patient will provide a narrative, but, it is not hard to imagine a rebellious teenager responding:

"Not much to say" [3].

Adding "Can you" to the beginning of a gentle command changes the dynamics. Of course, patients *can* tell you; it is a matter of *will* they tell you. I often see a trainee start an inquiry with "Can you..." when he feels tentative. Questioning regarding the quality of a situation or experience, a second category of questioning that appears open-ended but is not, takes the following form: starts with how; uses a form of the verb "to be"; and can be answered "fine" [3]. Again these questions only open up strongly engaged patients. Other patients answer "fine."

Clinician: How's your sleep?

Patient: Fine.

Of course, if a clinician does ask a shut-down patient the above question and gets that one word answer, he can simply follow it with:

"Okay. I didn't ask the question very well. I find that people mean different things by fine. Tell me about the different aspects of your sleep."

Thus the clinician substitutes a gentle command for the qualitative question.

LISTENING TO THE PATIENT'S COMMUNICATION

The patient's story, just like the physician's communication, can be understood on two levels – the social and the psychological. On the social level, the physician pays attention to the actual words of the patient [9].

Case: Mother: She has trouble breathing whenever she gets hot.

This mother seems to believe that getting warm or overheated precipitates her daughter's asthma. That is the social message. The psychological message underneath the words is revealed by nonverbal clues [9]. For example: if, in the above scenario, the mother adopted a hurried pace, raised her voice at the end of the sentence, and was fidgety in her chair, the psychological message might be:

"I'm worried about her."

By observing the patient's nonverbal messages, the clinician is in a better position to really understand the patient's perspective. Sometimes we describe this behavior as "listening to what is not said." Of course, the sense organs we use include our eyes as well as our ears.

TALKING WITH CHILDREN

The above techniques need to be modified when talking to children, especially young children, since they have cognitive and linguistic limitations that make them more vulnerable to anxiety in a strange situation like a clinical encounter.

The following strategies enhance engagement with children:

1. Explain the nature of the visit to children in words they can understand, so they know what is going to happen.

   "I am going to talk to you, Melissa, mommy and daddy about the pain in your tummy and going to school, so we can figure out a way for you to feel better and go to school."

2. Join with children by being friendly, maybe offering a toy or object to play with. Children between 6 months and 3 or 4 years of age, the age of separation anxiety, often respond best if given time to warm up before approaching them.

Case: Ericka is a 15-month old in for sick visit with cough and fever.

Before entering the exam room, Julie, a second year resident, makes a mental note of the child's age and presenting symptoms. She introduces herself and takes a seat on a stool 5–6 ft from mother and baby. She allows the baby plenty of time to adjust to this new stranger. While she is talking to mother, she has the baby sit on the mother's lap with no shirt or undershirt, enabling her to take an accurate respiratory rate, observes Ericka's work of breathing, her affect, and social interactions with mother. After Ericka appears comfortable with her, Julie offers her a toy in order to keep her occupied as she examines her.

3. Use concepts familiar with children of that age.

The clinician will be more successful in relating to children of preschool age through drawings and the use of words the preschooler has literally seen or experienced. For example, since a preschooler does not have a sophisticated or abstract understanding of cause and effect, the clinician can convey the idea of taking medicine to eradicate bacteria causing pneumonia by drawing bugs and showing the antibiotic medicine killing the bug [16].

A boy in elementary school with encoporesis understands the idea of strong muscles. He can be shown a drawing of dilated weak muscles in the bowel that need to be strengthened with his cooperation and regular bowel training.

4. When communicating with young children, make simple statements and ask questions with *concrete* references [17].

(To first grader)

Instead of: "Tell me about your teacher."

Say: "Does your teacher make it *fun?*"

5. Generous use of third-person technique. One way of adapting the third-person technique to young children is to tell them about a little girl or boy the clinician knows [17].

Clinician: I know a little girl who worries about her mommy when she is at school. Do you know any boys or girl like that girl?

Joan: Me. I'm like that

6. Avoid strict question and answer formats [17]. A conversational approach with echoing, tracking, empathic statements, and frequent affirmations helps children feel more comfortable in a strange clinical situation.

Thus, the language used with children is somewhere between the gentle commands noted above and the yes/no questions used by some adult clinicians

INTERNAL EXPERIENCE OF THE CLINICIAN

An easily overlooked task of the opening phase is for the clinician to check his own internal experience.

"What am I experiencing emotionally?"

When physicians recognize their own emotional state, they can use the feelings to guide them. This can lead to quite different responses by the clinician. Let us look at three examples:

Case: Mrs. Garfield is a 21-year-old mother who brings her two young children in for a clinic visit. She appears disorganized. The children are loud, running all around the room. The pediatric resident is aware of tenseness in his shoulders and chest. He is making himself anxious by telling himself that he will not be able to obtain an adequate history in the midst of this chaos. He believes that the attending will be disappointed, maybe even frustrated with him. Because this resident attends to the tenseness in his shoulders and chest and takes a moment to self-reflect, he recognizes his anxiety. He understands the root of it and knows he can manage it. He has a number of options. He enlists the help of Mrs. Garfield:

"Mrs. Garfield, I am having a difficulty. The kids are pretty active and I cannot hear you well enough to get a good history. How do you think we can handle this?"

He offers suggestions after Mrs. Garfield says she is open to them. Does she have someone to help? Would she control the children? Does she want to set up a play area in the room with an activity to interest the children? Would she like the resident to ask a staff member to help? Mrs. Garfield chooses the third option and it works well. He relaxes and takes the history.

Case: Mrs. Casey is a 25-year-old mother who brings her 4-year-old son, Larry, in for a yearly check up. Her main concern is that he has become aggressive and hyperactive. The pediatric resident obtains background information. He learns that Mrs. Casey's husband killed himself 6 months ago. Mrs. Casey moved to the area to be near her family and immediately went back to work. She is talking in a rapid, machine-gun like fashion. She does not appear sad but does look tense. As the pediatric resident takes a moment to self-reflect he notes a sense of sadness. He wonders if Mrs. Casey's hurried pace is covering her own sadness. He uses this information to respond to Mrs. Casey.

"Let me take a moment to think about what you just said. What you are saying is important."

The resident is quiet after making this statement. Mrs. Casey starts to sob, expressing her profound grief.

When patients make remarkable statements like the above one, it is important to slow the pace.

In the final example, a clinician, paying attention to her own internal experience, obtains information helpful for diagnosis.

Case: Misty is an outgoing, pleasant, and charming resident. She is receiving supervision regarding a family with a 1-month-old baby. She appears discouraged as she presents the family. She reports that the mother gave terse, almost argumentative responses to questions asking for routine information. When asked to consider what she was feeling emotionally, Misty replies that she was mildly annoyed. Since this is not her usual response to her patients, she considers that behaviors the mother exhibited might have influenced her; in addition, the mother might be inviting the same responses from other people. When asked by her mentor what could cause the mother to be argumentative, she lists several causes including postpartum depression. Misty screens for depression with the Edinburgh Postnatal Depression Scale. The score is in the positive range.

In all of the above examples, the resident stayed aware of his/her internal experience and used it to guide him/her. The final task of the opening phase is for the clinician to stay aware of the actual process of the interview.

PROCESS OF THE INTERVIEW

Two common process problems can make obtaining a valid data base very difficult.

- Patients who would not talk
- Patients who talk too much, often described as wandering

We can make effective adjustments if we recognize these interviewing styles early in the interview [3]. Shut-down interviews were discussed in Chap. 1: wandering interviews are the focus of Chap. 11. It is during the opening phase of the interview that the physician takes a brief look for any unusual problems. A patient may be confused and not understand the questions. Language barriers, very sick or sleepy patients, psychiatric illness, and drug abuse are other conditions that can profoundly interrupt the progression of the interview [3, 7]. The interviewer must address any of these issues *before* proceeding. For example, if the patient cannot give an accurate history, other sources of information will be necessary.

TRANSITIONING TO THE MIDDLE PHASE/ DISEASE-CENTERED PHASE

For most interviews, the clinician simply moves to the disease-centered and often more doctor-centered phase with a **transitional statement** [2].

> "Mrs. Green, let me summarize what I have heard you say so far ... Did I hear you right? ... Do you have any other concerns? ... Okay I'm now going to change direction and ask you more focused questions. Is that okay?"

Once any needed adjustments are made and the patient is fully engaged and talking actively, the interview moves into the second phase. The key goal of the second phase is to acquire a thorough and accurate data base (HPI, OAP[1], ROS, PMH, FH, Social History, [18]) in order to make good clinical decisions about the patient. The clinician's skill *guiding* the interview will receive its greatest challenge. Novice interviewers sometimes try so hard to be good listeners and engage the patient that they never take steps to influence the course of the interview. Once they realize they can influence the direction of the interview and still listen to the patient, they will be receptive to learning techniques for guiding the interview. Guiding the interview is particularly important when obtaining the history of present illness. Because of its importance, the next chapter will be exclusively devoted to the history of present illness.

References

1. Cole SA, Bird J (2000) The medical interview: the three function approach, 2nd edn. Mosby, Philadelphia
2. Smith RC (2002) Patient-centered interviewing: an evidence-based method, 2nd edn. Lippincott Williams and Wilkins, Philadelphia
3. Shea SC (1998) Psychiatric interviewing: the art of understanding: a practical guide for psychiatrics, psychologists, nurses, and other mental health professionals, 2nd edn. WB Saunders, Philadelphia
4. Korsch BM, Aley EF (1973) Pediatric interviewing techniques: current pediatric therapy. Sci Am 3:1–47
5. Platt FW, Gordon GH (2004) Field guide to the difficult interview, 2nd edn. Lippincott Williams and Wilkins, Baltimore, MD
6. Roter DL, Hall JA (2006) Doctors talking with patients/patients talking with doctors: improving communication in medical visits, 2nd edn. Praeger, Westport, CT
7. Platt FW, McMath JC (1979) Clinical hypocompetence: the interview. Ann Intern Med 91:898–902

---

[1]Other active problems – many of our patients, even children, have more than one current active problems.

8. Joines V (1997) Accessing the natural child as the key to redecision therapy. In: Lennox C (ed) Redecision therapy: a brief action-oriented approach. Jason Aronson, Northvale, NJ
9. Stewart I, Joines V (1987) T A today: a new introduction to transactional analysis. Lifespace, Chapel Hill, NC
10. Mishler EG (1984) The discourse of medicine: dialectics of medical interviews. Ablex, Norwood, NJ
11. Gould RK, Rothenberg MB (1973) The chronically ill child facing death: how can the pediatrician help. Clin Pediatr 12:447–449
12. Platt FW, Platt CM (1998) Empathy: a miracle or nothing at all? J Clin Outcomes Manage 5:30–33
13. Glasser H. Easley J (1998) Transforming the difficult child: the natural heart approach. Vaughan, Nashville, TN
14. Hall ET (1966) The hidden dimension. Doubleday, New York
15. Berne E (1966) Principles of group treatment. Grove, New York
16. Cline FW, Greene LC (2007) Parenting children with health issues. Love and Logic, Golden, CO
17. Sattler JM (1998) Clinical and forensic interviewing of children and families: guidelines for the mental health, education, pediatric, and child maltreatment fields. Jerome M. Sattler, San Diego, CA
18. Fortin AH, Dwamena FC, Smith RC (2005) Patient-centered interviewing. In: Tierney LM, Henderson MC (eds) The patient history: evidence-based approach. Lange Medical Books/McGraw Hill, New York

3
History of Present Illness

What else could it be? is a key safeguard against these errors in thinking: premature closure, framing effect, availability from recent experience, the bias that the hoof beats are horses and not zebras. … So a thinking doctor returns to language. 'Tell me the story again as if I never heard—what you felt, how it happened, when it happened.

Jerome Groopman, *How Doctors Think*

Eighteen seconds. Maybe 23 s. That's all the time an average patient has to tell his story before he is interrupted. Seventy percent of patients never get to finish their story [1, 2]. Why? The obvious answer: physicians feel rushed for time. However, that does not explain the 18 s fully. Why not interrupt after 2 s? I think the 18 s is a cursory attempt *to listen* to the patient before moving to the *real* task of the interview: gather symptom data needed for diagnosis. It is a false dichotomy. During the opening phase, the clinician listens to the patient *and* begins to gather psychosocial and biological data needed for accurate diagnosis (see Chap. 2). This takes 3–5 min to accomplish, not 18 s. The clinician listens to the patient *and* gathers data during the second phase of the interview as well. Only, the emphasis shifts to gathering the data that the patient does not spontaneously offer and that the clinician needs for accurate diagnosis.

All clinicians taking a history of present illness experience the tension of managing these two forces that seem to be in opposition. Over a century ago, William Osler taught young physicians to listen to the patient tell his story because he will "reveal the diagnosis [3]." Despite his emphasis on letting the patient talk, Osler fully acknowledged the other force – to gather specific details

J. Binder, *Pediatric Interviewing: A Practical, Relationship-Based Approach*, Current Clinical Practice, DOI 10.1007/978-1-60761-256-8_3, © Springer Science+Business Media, LLC 2010

about the symptom(s) even though the patient may be unaware of how essential they will be in making a correct diagnosis. I believe the clinician can resolve this tension by using an integrated, flexible interviewing style. In my experience, beginning interviewers often align with one side or the other. Either they adopt the strategy of asking the patient a succession of closed-ended, scripted, questions or they let the patient talk freely, without limits. Both techniques result in an incomplete history.

Case: Oscar is a 9-year-old boy with a cough. Tony and Martha are third year medical students. We join in as they are interviewing the mother.

TONY

Tony: What seems to be the trouble?

Mom: He has a cough.

Tony: How long has Oscar been coughing?

Mom: 4–5 days

Tony: Is the cough keeping him up at night?

Mom: Yes. The last two nights.

Tony: How many times has he been up?

Mom: 3–4 times.

Tony: Is the cough productive? Is he coughing up anything?

Mom: No.

Tony: Does he have vomiting or diarrhea?

Mom: No.

Tony: Does he have a runny nose?

Mom: No, but he had a sore throat last week.

Tony: Did he have any other symptoms with the sore throat?

Mom: He complained of his legs aching.

Tony: Has he had a fever?

Mom: He's had a fever for the last three days. It has gone up to 102.4

Tony: Does he have trouble breathing?

Mom: No.

Tony: Does he have a history of asthma?

Mom: None.

Tony: Have you given him anything for the cough?

Mom: Robitussin DM. It didn't help at all.

MARTHA

Martha: Tell me what the main difficulty has been.

Mom: Oscar has had a bad cough for 4–5 days.

Martha: Go on.

Mom: It's a congested cough.

Martha: What do you mean congested?

Mom: I can feel it in his chest

Martha: That sounds like it would be worrisome.

Mom: Yes. He's coughing hard and now he has chest pain.

Martha: Tell me more.

Mom: He can't sleep well.

Martha: He must be tired.

Mom: Yes. He's tired and cranky. He's not playing like usual.

Martha: Anything else?

Mom: Yes. I gave him Tylenol yesterday when his temperature was 102.4. It only came down to 101. Later, it went back up and I gave it again.

Martha: Did that help?

Mom: Not much.

Martha: I see.

Both Tony and Martha clearly have emerging interviewing skills. Tony is eliciting specific details and quantifying data. Martha is tracking with mom, empathizing with her, and establishing a strong engagement. Their strategies have notable pitfalls. Tony did not encourage the mother to talk freely and missed important data (e.g. chest pain). Martha did not carefully inquire about a number of dimensions of the cough, including associated symptoms. She missed that the illness began with a sore throat, headache, and muscular achiness for several days before onset of cough in a classic presentation of *Mycoplasm pneumoniae* infection. It is interesting to note that Tony did begin with one open-ended question. Clinicians almost always do begin with such a question, perhaps "What can we do for you today?" or "What seems to be the trouble?" But the high-control interviewer who is addicted to "yes–no" sorts of inquiry quickly abandons that open-ended approach. Both students had incomplete data.

The ability of the diagnostician to make the right diagnosis is dependent on the interviewer obtaining a full and accurate history. Recent research has confirmed that jumping to conclusions is a common cause of misdiagnosis. And, misdiagnosis is a leading cause of clinical error [4]. Occasionally, a physician recognizes a classic pattern of symptoms that is highly suggestive of one diagnosis (e.g. chronic honking cough that disappears with sleep and the diagnosis of a psychogenic cough). Much more often, clinical practice requires the rational application of the principles of epidemiology and clinical medicine to formulate a clear differential diagnosis. The *myth*: Making the correct diagnosis is a result of a clever *hunch*.

PLAN FOR HPI

Tony and Martha need a template describing a method for gathering all the data that would support making an accurate diagnosis. These two students must first have a clear concept of how to explore a symptom. William Morgan and George Engel emphasized the importance of **carefully, methodically, and precisely** investigating the seven dimensions of any symptom in their classic text: The Clinical Approach to the Patient [5]. The following is a thumbnail sketch of the *seven* dimensions.

Location and radiation – an attempt to obtain a precise description is made. An area of pain may be small or large, superficial or deep, radiate or not. (Patients can be asked to point to their pain). The key questions have to do with "Where is it?" and "Where else?" The description of the location and radiation can help the clinician form hypotheses [5].

> Ex: Visceral pain is usually poorly localized because of the distribution of nocicepters [6].

Chronology: The chronology provides the structure for the other six dimensions of the patient's story. It is important to establish the time of onset, duration, intervals, and course using calendar time. If the patient can use specific landmarks like a birthday or holiday, confidence in the accuracy of the time line is increased. All time intervals need to be accounted for. If the symptoms are episodic, a recent, specific example is examined and the long-term course defined, placing individual episodes as they have occurred over the months or years. Patients are asked: "Then what happened?" Obtaining all relevant details helps the interviewer understand the **big picture** [5]. It can be very helpful to know why the family decided to come at this time. Have the symptoms persisted too long or increased in severity? Did they begin to worry?

Tony and Martha's patient, Oscar, presented with fever, sore throat, headache, and myalgia for days before he developed a persistent cough that interfered with his sleep, leading mom to make an appointment for a sick visit.

Neither student, Martha or Tony, reconstructed the *chronology* of the symptoms carefully in the case at the beginning of the chapter.

Quality – This can be ascertained simply by asking what the symptom feels like. Most patients are eager to describe the qualities of the symptom and use highly metaphorical language. Unfortunately, the quality of a symptom is not as helpful diagnostically as we would like. If the patient does not describe the symptom, one strategy is to give them choices [7]:

"Is the pain dull, aching, sharp, crushing,…?"

The problem with that strategy is that a patient may attempt to fit his symptom into one of the categories, instead of describing his symptom in his own terms. Sometimes, a patient who has difficulty describing a symptom will respond to being asked a second time and waiting for a reply:

"So, how would you describe the pain?"

If a patient does not fill in the details with this second inquiry, specific choices can then be offered. One of the choices may be through comparison. A symptom is often characterized by comparison [5]. (e.g. The cough of croup sounds like the bark of a seal). The clinician establishes the quality of a symptom before asking about the quantitative aspects of a symptom, in order to understand what the patient/parent is quantifying. Novice interviewers have a tendency to ask about quantity first [8].

Quantity – A number of features must be considered in this category: type of onset, intensity of symptom, *degree of functional impairment*, frequency, size, … (see Table 3.1). Precision is important. Vague answers like "not much" are followed up with further questioning. Functional impairment can be evaluated by having the patient describe his activities over a specific recent day. This is likely to provide better details then a *typical* day [5].

TABLE 3.1. The seven descriptors of symptoms

Location and radiation
(1) Precise location
(2) Deep or superficial
(3) Specific or diffuse

Chronology and timing – course of individual symptom over time
   Time of onset of symptom and intervals between its occurrence
   Duration of symptom
   Periodicity and frequency of symptom
   Course of symptom
   (a) Short term
   (b) Long term

Quality
(1) Usual descriptors
(2) Unusual descriptors

Quantification
(1) Type of onset
(2) Intensity or severity
(3) Impairment or disability
(4) Numerical description
   (a) Number of events
   (b) Size
   (c) Volume

Setting

Moderating factors
(1) Precipitants or aggravating factors
(2) Relieving factors

Associated symptoms (adapted from patient-centered interviewing by
Robert C. Smith)

> "Walk me through yesterday with Oscar. Start when he got
> up in the morning."

Setting – Exploring what the patient was doing and where he
was as the symptoms developed can help characterize a symptom
as well as give a window into the life of the patient. Often, this
information is obtained during the patient's initial description of
his symptoms. At other times the clinician must ask about recent
events such as travel [5].

> "Tell me what Oscar was doing and where he was around
> the time he became ill?"

Aggravating/Alleviating Factors – A symptom can be influenced by
activities such as eating, exercising, and sleeping. The patient is asked
about any factor that appears to help or worsen the condition [5].

> "Tell me anything that seems to aggravate or bring on the pain."

If the patient found that hard to answer, a clinician might try:

> "Tell me what you have found you have to avoid to not make the pain reappear or get worse."

Once the patient has had a chance to respond to this open-ended inquiry, he can be asked about specific factors that he may be unaware are related to his symptoms:

> "Have you noticed any effect of eating chocolate or cheese on your headaches?"

Similarly some patients will respond to your questions ("Tell me anything that lessens the pain") about alleviating factors with "Nothing, Doctor. That's why I've come to you." But even then they may be helpful if you asked:

> "What do you find yourself doing after you get this symptom."

Associated Symptoms – Malfunction of a given organ usually expresses itself with other symptoms that involve that organ, as well as related systemic or general effects. Experienced clinicians are familiar with common symptom groupings. *They form hypotheses based on the grouping of symptoms.* That is how they *organize* their history of present illness [5]. A toddler with intermittent abdominal pain, vomiting, and blood in the stools suggests the possibility of intussusception.

Young clinicians need an organizing principle until they gain experience and knowledge and can generate hypotheses. That principle is *timing*. Symptoms are grouped according to their time of occurrence. The time line becomes their organizing principle. This is the foundation of the template we will teach Tony and Martha. It is the structure proposed by Robert Smith in *Patient-Centered Interviewing* [7].

TEMPLATE FOR GATHERING DATA

The first task is for the interviewer to obtain the *chief complaint* (most pressing symptom), *any other major symptoms*, their time of onset, and a rough time line [7].

Case: A 3-year-old with hematuria, whose mother also mentions mild diarrhea for 2 days.

The clinician inquires, in detail, about the seven cardinal features of the main symptom (hematuria) using a chronological framework. The clinician asks specifically for details in the seven descriptors that parent has not already mentioned during the initial open-ended exploration of the symptom. The clinician asks about the presence or absence of symptoms from the review of systems of the body system involved (urinary – dysuria, urgency, loss of bladder control, abdominal pain, vomiting, ...). If a symptom suggests more than one body system then they are all explored [7].

Other symptoms (diarrhea), whether initially mentioned by the patient or uncovered later, are explored. Again, the seven cardinal features are carved out and the body system involved – gastrointestinal – is expanded (symptoms of vomiting, abdominal pain, appetite, etc.). If the timing is similar to the main symptom, a more *efficient* way to develop a second symptom is to explore it simultaneously with the main symptom [7].

> "Tell me about the blood in the urine, the diarrhea and other symptoms, starting from the beginning."

The clinician will still need to ask for individual characteristics of each symptom as she expands the descriptors of quality, quantity, and occasionally moderating factors.

> "What is the frequency of the diarrhea?"

Questions about any effect on general health are asked, such as ***affect, activity level, appetite, fever, pain, and change in weight*** [7]. Then the clinician inquires about *nonsymptom* data. Nonsymptom data include previous diagnoses, medications, and hospitalizations. These can include any *relevant* data from the *past medical history, social history, family history, and travel history*. Sometimes which material is relevant is not clear until further in the interview [7].

Some clinicians gather nonsymptom data first, especially with patients who have had extensive medical evaluations and treatment in the past. It is important that these clinicians then return and obtain symptom data. Symptoms can be viewed as *primary* data, facts known to the patient. The nonsymptom data tend to be more a matter of hearsay, thus not really known to the patient. If one relies on these nonprimary data, past mistakes in diagnosis get perpetuated.

Once the clinician has clarified and developed the symptoms, along with the secondary data, and placed them along a time line, she has the data needed for disease diagnosis. These are the data Martha and Tony must gather.

PROCESS
Initially, Tony and Martha will need to scan for the possibility of associated symptoms extensively. If a patient presents with a headache, they will need to thoroughly scan from both the neurological and HEENT review of systems, since headaches can result from

conditions in both areas [visual changes, weakness or sensory changes on one side, mental status changes, speech difficulties, vomiting, night awakening, dental pain, nasal stuffiness, cough (sinusitis), pain with jaw motion, etc.] [7].Once they have all the data they will formulate a differential diagnosis. This inductive method works. However, it is time consuming. Expert diagnosticians tend to start developing theories very early and use further data to substantiate their theories [9]. With time and experience, these young clinicians will not inquire about every possible symptom. They will begin to form hypotheses about what is causing the patient's symptoms. They will ask questions related to those hypotheses and scan briefly for other possibilities [10].

Questions are asked that shorten the list as the clinician moves from the *general to the specific*. The hazard of this shortcut approach is too quickly making a specific diagnosis, potentially leaving out alternative diagnoses for consideration all together [11]. The amount of scanning will be based on what the patient reveals. If the patient has recurrent headaches for 2 years with features of tension headaches, she might scan the neurological review of systems with a few general questions (e.g. visual changes, weakness, vomiting) to ensure that she is not missing the diagnosis. Conversely, if a child persists with a continuous, progressive headache for a month, she will fully scan the neurological system because of the possibility of a central nervous system lesion and/or increased intracranial pressure. *Beginning interviewers are more likely to obtain a complete data base if they follow the same order of asking about symptom descriptors each time so they don't leave out any dimensions.*

THE WEAVE

Some patients will provide much of the data needed for symptom description simply through repeated open invitations to talk about their symptoms. Other patients will need many focused questions to fully carve their symptoms. One useful approach for either type of patient is the **weave**. The clinician uses a gentle command whenever a new topic (e.g. factors that exacerbate the symptom) is introduced **and** whenever a patient responds positively to an inquiry (e.g. Has his breathing been affected?). She follows those open-ended inquiries with focused questions to gather details not spontaneously offered by the patient. The clinician **weaves** back and forth between open-ended and closed ended inquiries, depending on the patient's response.

Case: A clinician exploring the *modifying* descriptor of the symptom of cough.

Clinician:	Have you noticed anything that makes the cough worse
Parent:	I haven't noticed.
Clinician:	How about any change at night.
Parent:	Yes, he coughs more when he lies down. It kept him up last night.
Clinician:	Tell me about that. (Clinician moves back to open-ended inquiry after hearing a positive response to her closed-ended question.)
Parent:	He woke up at 2 A.M. and was coughing. He was up for an hour and one-half before I was able to help him settle down. I rocked him back to sleep. Then he woke up this morning at 5 A.M. coughing and wheezing. I gave him his inhaler and he was able to breathe easier and go back to sleep. He is exhausted. I'm pretty tired myself.
Clinician:	It does sound tiring.
Parent:	Yeah, we're both tired today.
Clinician:	How has it affected him during the daytime. (Clinician moves back to a focused inquiry to fully carve out the sub region, quantity, which includes impact on child's functioning.)

Platt and Gordon describe the weaving process:

> "The challenge is to put the patient on the right track, then to sit back and let him tell us what we need to hear. On the other hand, we have a lot to do too. We are seeking a clear understanding of the specific details, trying to translate the patient's story into medical data...Throughout the conversation there must be a balance between the doctor's inquiry and the patient's narrative" [12].

Roter and Hall demonstrated the connection between interviewing style and data collection in a seminal study in 1987. Physicians obtained more relevant information by a ratio of 2:1, when they asked open-ended rather than closed-ended questions. Open-ended questions invited the patients to elaborate. Closed-ended questions restricted patient's responses [13]. Practicing physicians use many more closed-ended than open-ended questions. Their belief is that closed-ended questions are more efficient once the diagnosis have begun to be narrowed. This study contradicts that belief. Although closed-ended questions are essential for obtaining specific details left out by the patient, a greater use of open-ended questions improves data collection. A blend of open and closed-ended questions throughout appears optimal for data collection [13]. In the long run, the most *efficient* interviewing strategies are those that get the patient to talk. Elmer Holzinger, designated a master-clinician at the University of Pittsburgh for his excellence in teaching medical students [14], illustrates this point with the following story (based on a conversation in the spring of 2006). A patient being interviewed by a student incidentally mentions he couldn't finish his meals. Before the patient could tell the student his jaw muscles became fatigued, the student asked: "Is it painful?" By asking for a specific detail instead of having the patient elaborate, he prevented the patient from telling him the diagnosis.

Sackett et al. recommended two resources for clinicians wishing to increase the power of the focused questions they ask during the HPI: read the literature and seek expert consultation regarding the sensitivity and specificity of a given question with regard to diagnosing a clinical condition [9]. A recent example from the journal, Neurology, illustrates this beautifully. Video EEG recording was utilized. Eye-opening and closing were observed and recorded during seizures. One-hundred fifty two of the 156 patients with epileptic seizures opened their eyes. Fifty out of 52 patients with psychogenetic nonepileptic seizures closed their eyes during the seizure. Asking about eye opening and closing has a very good discriminatory power in differentiating these two conditions [15]. However, most conditions can present in such a variety of ways that one question will neither make nor eliminate a diagnosis [10]. *The clinician must look at the big picture.*

THE BIG PICTURE

The discriminatory power of a question can vary remarkably with the clinical context, the other symptoms that are associated with an index symptom. The clinician attempts to base questions on the *underlying physiology*. Uncovering mild early morning intraorbital puffiness in the context of a prolonged thick nasal discharge, wet cough, halitosis, and mildly decreased activity in a toddler suggests an ethmoid sinusitis, whereas bilateral periorbital edema in the context of an increasing abdominal girth secondary to ascites is classic for the nephrotic syndrome.

The context includes epidemiological factors such as the patient's age and gender. These factors can affect the likelihood of a specific diagnosis [16]. A toddler with crampy abdominal pain and bloody stools is much more likely to have intussusception than a school-aged child with abdominal pain and bloody stools [17]. A very young child with signs of appendicitis, but no anorexia, may very well have appendicitis. *Only* 60–70% of *very young* children with appendicitis have anorexia [18]. Anorexia is a more sensitive indicator of appendicitis in older children. The finding that the absence of anorexia does not *rule out* the diagnosis of appendicitis in very young children highlights an important principle.

The absence of a clinical finding with high sensitivity is useful for excluding diagnosis; the presence of a clinical finding with high specificity is useful for confirming diagnosis [16].

REAL PATIENTS

So far, we have assumed that gathering the clinical history is straightforward. Any trainee will attest to the fact that real live patients often are more complex. For example, a clinician may be faced with any of the following:

- A patient presents with a vague complaint that is not a symptom from the review of symptoms. (e.g. wiped out; dizzy; funny smelly urine; trouble breathing...) [7].
- The patient presents numerous symptoms that seem disconnected (e.g. dysuria, heartburn, fever, chronic cough and congestion, picky eater).
- The patient has one or more chronic conditions

    An 11-year-old child with diabetes mellitus presents with vomiting. Is it related to the diabetes and its treatment or is a separate illness?

- The patient has symptoms suggestive of a functional condition (e.g. abdominal pain only on school days).

    Luckily, there are excellent options available for trainees like Tony and Martha, who are learning to *organize* these more complex interviews. The preceptor tells Tony and Martha that she has found the following strategies increase her efficiency while managing complex interviews.

1. Turn any nonsymptom complaint into a symptom – from the review of symptoms.

    Open with a gentle command and use closed-ended questions to clarify.

    Patient: I feel dizzy (unclear diagnosis)

    Physician: Tell me what you mean by dizzy.

    Patient: I feel unsteady.

Physician: Tell me more about it.

Patient: I feel like I might fall.

Physician: Do you get a sensation of movement, like you just stepped off a merry-go-round or do you feel light-headed, like you might faint? [7]

Patient: It's more like I'm spinning, or moving.

This patient has vertigo, which has a different meaning to the clinician than light headedness. Another parent may report a "cold," thus naming her own self-diagnosis or one given to her by anther person, or may report "trouble breathing" that seems to be a symptom but indeed might mean anything from dyspnea to a stuffy nose. It is a good practice to clarify what a parent means even when they refer to a symptom from the review of symptoms: e.g. weakness; diarrhea [8]. They may not be using the term as you define it medically.

2. Take one problem at a time when the symptoms appear totally unrelated [8].

   "Let's take these problems one at time. What do you think is the main difficulty?"

3. If a problem is clearly unrelated to the HPI and belongs either in the other active problems section or perhaps even later in the review of symptoms, this can be stated [8]:

   "It is important for me to obtain a clear picture of the symptoms that Nancy has experienced recently. We will cover those other symptoms a little later. Is that Okay?"

Note: When a clinician asks the patient if he has any other problems during the first phase of the interview and gives him a chance to talk about these problems (medical or personal), she avoids the occasional *positive review of systems* later in the interview. Use of questions such as "What else?" tends to empty the review of systems [19]. Nothing current and important should surface later on if the ROS has been emptied out in the early phases of the interview.

4. Summarize the history at the conclusion of characterizing the current somatic symptoms, then transition to the past medical history to inquire about any chronic illness [8].The same approach can be used to get the social history when the diagnosis of a functional condition is part of the differential diagnosis.

   "So let me see if I have it right. Sounds like Shania has had episodes of abdominal pain lasting 30–60 minutes and occurring before school and in the evening. This has been going for a month. She has no other symptoms, is growing well and staying active. Yes? I would like to now shift gears and ask about school and her relationships with family and friends."

Tony and Martha are appreciative of these options. They liked the idea of summarizing to guide the interview to a new topic. They are curious about other ways of guiding the interview to a new area, without discouraging the patient from telling her story.

INTERVIEWING STYLE

Interviewing *style* determines whether the patient will provide a full and complete data base [20]. A decade after Roter and Hall's study, Shea asserted that *maintaining* a strong engagement throughout the history of present illness activates a patient. A solid engagement is maintained by tracking and empathy, as well as by conversational-style transitional or bridging techniques. A patient is not likely to share all relevant information when the physician uses a cold, hurried "meet-the press" style such as Tony did. This next example was reported by Barbara Korsch.

Mother: Then for the last two days he's been vomiting, and this morning started...

Doctor: (Interrupting) When did the diarrhea start?

Mother: This morning. About four times he vomited.

Doctor: Okay. How long has he had the running nose? Any fever?

Mother: Oh, just a little bit, and he is unable to keep anything in his stomach.

Doctor: All right. Has he been urinating today? [21]

The interviewer is missing data with regard to the vomiting. She is also missing data with regard to mom's anxiety about the vomiting. The underlying message to the mother is

What you have to say is not important.

We can maintain a strong engagement, much like a conversation between friends. This is not meant to imply that an effective physician–patient relationship is simply a friendly relationship. Effective care depends on taking a biopsychosocial approach and constructing the meaning of illness through the interview with the patient [22]. A friendly relationship may improve the quality of the relationship, but this is not sufficient to provide effective care. Nonetheless, it is instructive to analyze a conversation between friends:

- One person is activated to talk about a topic.
- The other friend is interested, listens actively, and tracks with the friend (recall that tracking refers to the process of commenting or asking a question about what the person just said).
- Friends usually talk about a topic until it is *finished*.
- Once a topic is completed, they make a smooth transition to the next topic [20].

In a parallel manner to the conversation between friends, the well-engaged clinician

- Makes generous use of gentle commands and open-ended questions to activate a patient and enhance engagement, both at the beginning and throughout the exploration of a topic.
- Tracks with the patient (formulates questions based on what the patient just said).
- Stays with the topic before moving on to the next topic. This conveys a message to the patient that the clinician is being careful and thorough.
- Once a topic is completed, a smooth transition is made to the next topic. Shea called topic areas **"*regions*"** and transition statements **"*gates*"** [20]. Mishler used the term **"*tie*"** for transitions [22]. Knowledge of gates or ties gives the clinician a way to **guide** the patient through the HPI and maintain a conversation-style interview.

GATES

Spontaneous gate – An important decision the clinician must make is how to respond to the patient's spontaneous movement to a new subject before the clinician feels completed with the previous subject. Some clinicians let the patient talk a bit in order to determine whether *to follow* the patient through the spontaneous gate. I think that *once the opening of the interview is complete*, 90% of the time it is a better idea to immediately return to the first topic. If the patient expresses emotion or moves to a sensitive topic, such as suicide, I believe the clinician should follow the patient's lead. In these instances the clinician **weaves** back and forth. Otherwise, the clinician returns to the original topic by asking a question in the first subregion, not tracking to the next subregion:

Case: Mother just left subregion of quality of cough to mention she gave Tylenol.

> "I'd like you to go back for a moment. You said the cough was harsh. Tell me more about what it sounds like."

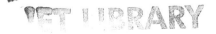

Alternatively, the clinician can acknowledge what the patient just said and let her know she will return to that topic, but stay with the initial topic (subregion) [20].

Physician: Tell me about the cough.

Mother: It's harsh.

Physician: Say more.

Mother: Well. She has chest pain and fever with it. The pain is on the left side (spontaneous movement to a new topic).

Physician: That's important. We will come back to the pain. First, tell me more about what the cough sounds like.

Comment: (Physician does not follow patient through the spontaneous gate.)

Mother: She had a cold for several days. She developed a mild cough that sounded like she had mucous in her throat.

Physician: And now?

Mother: It sounds dry and harsh. I think it is her chest.

Comment: The physician goes on to explore other cardinal features of the cough. He then returns to associated symptoms with a referred gate.

Physician: A minute ago you mentioned chest pain. Start at the beginning and tell me about it.

This approach is based on the assumption that it is more *time efficient* to stay in a subregion, instead of going back and forth [20]. In addition, it is easier to remember what questions (details) need to be asked when they are *blocked* in memory. This can also contribute to patient's sense of physician's expertise when she sees that the clinician knows what to ask. The clinicians can come back to this area later in the interview using a referred gate or summarizing technique.

> "Earlier you said he had chest pain. Tell me more about that." (referred gate)

Because we want to save some items for later, we need a mental parking place, a sorted list of items we plan to ask about later on. Many students wonder about note keeping. We suggest that a scratch pad be used to jot down words that remind us of topics we want to return to later, topics that have been suggested by the history-giver (parent or child) or that we thought of ourselves during the interview. Thus, the this clinician might jot down "chest pain" to aid in remembering that we want to return to that topic shortly but need not be diverted to do it right now. When the clinician feels finished with a topic area (subregion), she has a number of options for transitioning the interview to the next region or subregion. These techniques solidify the conversational feel of the history and help keep the patient activated.

Transition statements that are particularly helpful in going from one region or subregion to another when obtaining a history of present illnesses are implied, natural, and referred gates, the third person technique, and summarization.

Implied Gate – the interviewer simply moves the interviewee to a new topic that appears to generally be related to the first topic [20]. In the following example, the interviewer moves from the HPI subregion of severity (quantity) to associated symptoms of general health.

Parent:	The abdominal pain seems severe. He is crying with pain.
Physician:	I see. Tell me what his activity has been like.
Parent:	Ah. He hasn't played at all today. He is just lying on the couch and watching TV.
Physician:	How has his overall mood been today?
Parent:	He has been whiny.
Physician:	What other symptoms have you noticed?
Parent:	He hasn't eaten a bite. He is drinking Seven-Up.

Natural gate – The natural gate consists of two parts, a cue statement made by the patient or parent and a transitional question by the interviewer. When done well the interviewee "will feel that the conversation is flowing from his own speech, as indeed it is. Such a transition seems both natural and caring to the interviewee" ([20], p. 116).

This physician uses a natural gate to guide the HPI from describing the quantity dimensions of a cough to the associated systemic symptoms.

Parent:	He has a cough, especially at night.
Physician:	Is the cough waking him up?
Parent:	Once or twice at night (cue statement).

Physician:	Is this having any effect on his energy level? (transitional statement)
Parent:	Maybe a little.
Physician:	Tell me about his activity and play today.

Referred gate – A clinician refers back to an earlier statement by the patient and uses that statement to move to a new topic [20].

Parent:	I think the cough is hurting his throat.
Pediatrician:	What makes you think his throat is hurting?
Parent:	He won't eat.
Pediatrician:	I see. Earlier you said his belly was hurting. Tell me more about that. (Referred gate)
Parent:	Well he seems to be cramping up before he has a bowel movement.

The third person technique, an interesting corollary of the referred gate, refers to the general category of people presenting with this symptom. Instead of referring back to a specific statement made by a particular patient, the third person technique is used to ask questions about features of the symptom that other patients have experienced [23].

Parent:	Jonathan's abdominal pain really seems to be bothering him. He won't eat breakfast.
Physician:	Tell me more.
Parent:	He says his stomach hurts and that he is not hungry.
Physician:	Lots of children who have abdominal pain in the morning tend to be sensitive kids and worry. Is that true for Jonathan? (third person technique).
Parent:	Yes, it is.
Physician:	Tell me about his worrying.
Comment:	This tool gives the interviewer leverage to smoothly move the interview in the direction she would like to go.

Summarization helps the clinician recap essential features of what the patient has so far said [8]. It eases transition from one topic (subregion) to the next.

Physician:	Let me see if I have heard you right. The cough is frequent over the last two days, occurring almost

	hourly at night and waking Johnny from his sleep. He is also having spasms of coughing, did I get it right?
Parent:	Yes.
Physician:	Now tell me anything that seems to bring on the cough.

As Tony and Martha experiment with using the transitional statements, they may find several that fit their style. It is not important for them to use them all in each interview. In fact, as they begin their interviewing careers they are likely to limit themselves to **implied gates and summarization**. Transitioning by summarizing gives an uncertain interviewer time to think about which direction to take next. The clinician who practices incorporating **referred and natural gates** into her interviews will add flexibility and richness.

Let us turn to a case example. Observe these principles being applied during the HPI of a 14-year-old girl with 2-week history of chest pain. Her name is Amanda.

HPI 14-YEAR-OLD GIRL WITH CHEST PAIN

Pediatrician:	Tell me about your chest pain and everything else about your illness. (gentle command)
Amanda:	My chest really hurts. Right here. (Patient points to sternum). (location)
Pediatrician:	It's very painful. And it hurts right in the middle of your chest.
Amanda:	Yes. (Patient appears apprehensive)
Pediatrician:	Anywhere else?
Amanda:	No
Pediatrician:	Why don't you start from the beginning and tell me about your chest pain. (gentle command)
Amanda:	Well, it started two weeks ago when I was in class at school. I'm coughing; I don't feel good. (context)
Comment:	It is less than one minute into the interview. The clinician postpones getting the personal story to a later time. The clinician recognizes a pattern: acute and increasing chest pain associated with the systemic symptoms of not feeling "good." This is suggestive of a cardiac or pulmonary etiology. The other major causes of chest pain in children— functional, musculoskeletal, gastrointestinal— are unlikely with this

presentation. Musculoskeletal causes don't typically get worse over the time course of two weeks or become associated with systemic symptoms. The same is true for functional and gastrointestinal complaints which frequently are recurrent. So the first non-specific hypothesis of this clinician is: this is a cardiac or pulmonary condition. The clinician has a choice at this pivot point. The patient has spontaneously entered a sub region of associated symptoms ("not feeling good"). The clinician elects not to follow the patient into that sub region, but rather to stay and fully explore the characteristics of the chest pain itself, starting with the quality of the pain.

Pediatrician:	So really not feeling good and coughing. Well, let's go back and tell me what the pain has been like. (gentle command)
Amanda:	It's there all the time. And my back hurts too.
Pediatrician:	Say more about what it feels like.
Amanda:	My chest feels heavy. And the pain is sharp. (quality)
Pediatrician:	How do you mean sharp.
Amanda:	Like I'm being stabbed with a knife.
Comment:	The clinician now moves to quantity, another cardinal dimension of the symptom, with a referred gate.
Pediatrician:	Earlier you said the pain has been present for two weeks and is getting more painful. Tell me more about that. Start with how it started.
Amanda:	It came on one afternoon during algebra class. It stayed that way until two days ago. The day before yesterday it became even worse. It just won't ease up.
Pediatrician:	On a scale of one to ten, with ten being the worst pain you have experienced, how painful would you rate it?
Amanda:	A nine or ten.
Pediatrician:	Wow, that sounds bad. Have you found anything that makes it feel better? (modifying factors)
Amanda:	At first, when I lied down. Now I would rather sit up.

Pediatrician:	What happens when you lie down? (An open-ended question encourages the patient to make any number of responses vs. the restriction imposed by a yes/no question.)
Amanda:	I'm not comfortable. It is easier to breathe sitting up.
Pediatrician:	So your position affects your breathing? How about taking a deep breath. Does that affect the pain?
Amanda:	I haven't noticed that.
Pediatrician:	Have you noticed anything that does make it worse?
Amanda:	Walking, I can barely walk around the house.
Pediatrician:	What happens? (open-ended questions)
Amanda:	I get short of breath and feel dizzy.
Pediatrician:	Let me see if I have everything right so far. You have had chest pain for two weeks. It's a heavy feeling, sometimes sharp and it is a severe pain. Your position seems to affect it. In addition, you don't feel good and have had trouble just walking around because you get short of breath. And, you started coughing. (summarization)
Amanda:	Yes.
Comment:	The clinician is leaning toward a cardiac cause, even though statistically it is infrequent. She wants to eliminate pulmonary causes, if she can, before more fully exploring cardiovascular conditions. She mentally reviews common and important pulmonary causes of chest pain to organize her thinking (asthma, pneumonia, pleural effusions, pneumothorax/pneumo-mediastinum, pulmonary embolus).
Pediatrician:	Earlier you mentioned you were coughing. (referred gate)
Amanda:	Yes, I have been.
Pediatrician:	Tell me more about the cough. (weaving)
Amanda:	It's deep. It started a couple of days ago. Sometimes I vomit because I'm coughing.
Pediatrician:	How many times have you vomited?

Amanda: Two times.

Pediatrician: Have you coughed up any mucous?

Amanda: No.

Pediatrician: Have you had any fever with the cough? (implied gate)

Amanda: No, I haven't.

Comment: The presence of a productive sounding cough is compatible with pulmonary and cardiac conditions. It is imperative to ask questions that discriminate between these two categories. In this case, the onset of the cough came well after the onset of chest pain. Furthermore, she has experienced "dizziness" with very limited physical activity. The cough was most likely due to cardiac condition. The pediatrician decides to use a natural gate to organize his inquiry into associated symptoms.

Pediatrician: Is the cough keeping you up at night?

Amanda: Sometimes.

Pediatrician: Tell me about that. (weaving)

Amanda: I woke up a couple times last night and the night before. It's not really a bad cough, but it takes me awhile to get back to sleep. My mom gave me some medicine to help. (cue statement)

Pediatrician: Has this trouble sleeping interfered with your energy level? (natural gate – transitional question)

Amanda: Yes, I haven't rested well.

Pediatrician: Tell me about your energy level over the last 1–2 days. (gentle command)

Amanda: I just lie down and watch TV. I can't concentrate to read.

Pediatrician: Has your appetite been affected? (implied gate)

Amanda: Yes. I'm not very hungry.

Pediatrician: And your mood? (implied gate)

Amanda: I'm real worried.

Pediatrician: What are you most worried about? (asking for her self-diagnosis)

Amanda:	My heart.
Pediatrician:	What specifically about your heart concerns you?
Amanda:	I know heart disease is serious.
Pediatrician:	That's got to be frightening. When I finish your evaluation we will talk about this worry.
Pediatrician:	Have you noticed your heart racing?
Amanda:	It beats real fast when I stand up.
Pediatrician:	Is it uncomfortable?
Amanda:	Not really. It just feels a little weird.
Pediatrician:	Let me check with you again to make sure I have heard everything correctly. You have had chest pain for two weeks. It is now severe and feels heavy and sharp at times. You don't feel good: your appetite is down. You started with a cough several days ago and are sleeping poorly. You are having trouble being active because you get short of breath and are tired. You are naturally worried about all this and wonder if something is wrong with your heart. (summarization)
Amanda:	Yes, I'm worried. My heart beats fast

Pediatrician: As soon as I finish checking you out I will talk to you and mom about what all this means. Earlier you had mentioned you felt dizzy. Tell me about that. (referred gate)

Amanda:	I feel very lightheaded.
Pediatrician:	Have you actually passed out?

Amanda: I almost passed out yesterday, when I was walking to the bathroom. That's the only time.

Comment: The pediatrician has inquired about associated symptoms, including general health functioning maintaining a chronological framework. He will now ask for non symptom data: any previous medical diagnosis, work up, or treatment of this condition; as well as, information from the past medical history, family history, or social history that might be relevant (e.g. history of using cardiotoxic medication, family history of cardiac disease etc.)

In this annotated interview, the clinician gathered the information she needed to make a solid differential diagnosis. At the

TABLE 3.2. Structure for obtaining the history of present illness

Obtain chief complaint, other major symptoms, and rough time course (during the patient-centered phase of the interview). The more you learn by open inquiry, the less you will have to probe for later on. Asking the patient to "tell me about it" will often uncover the bulk of the needed data and speed up the interview. Paradoxically, neophyte interviewers often believe that they will get more data by going right to narrow focused questioning. Almost certainly a mistake.

Ask for details of the seven cardinal features of the main symptom, including associated symptoms in the body system (e.g. genitourinary) or systems involved with the symptom (e.g. hematuria).

Do the same for other symptoms – can be done concurrently with main symptom if time lines are parallel.

Ask about effects on general health.

Obtain relevant nonsymptom data.

TABLE 3.3. Components of the history of present illness

Goal: Formulate solid differential diagnosis while maintaining strong engagement as patient tells his *story*

Content: Location; *timing and chronology*; characteristics or quality of the symptoms; quantity; context; modifying factors; associated symptoms; nonsymptom data.

Style: Conversational expansion
    Weave between open-ended statements and focused questions, depending on the patient's response/gentle commands to explore positive responses
    Guide the interview to subregions through the use of transitional statements
    Focused questions to obtain missing details

Macro strategy:
    Move from a short list of non-specific hypotheses to short list of specific hypotheses
    Questions asked to positively support a diagnosis are supplemental by questions that *discriminate* between conditions
    Look at the big picture

same time, she maintained engagement with the patient by tracking with the patient, expressing empathic statements, uncovering the patient's self diagnosis, and making the interview into a conversation. Simultaneously, she gently guided the interview using implied, natural, and referred transition statements. This enabled her to obtain all the data she needed. She used a number of gentle commands even as she went from general to more specific hypotheses. This allowed the patient to tell her *story*. Based on the time course, severity, progression of the pain and associated symptoms of dyspnea on exertion, fatigue, lightheadedness, and heart "racing," the clinician placed cardiomyopathy as her working diagnosis. Pericarditis was only an alternative diagnosis because of the lack of pleuritic pain, history of fever or viral symptoms. She thought a tachyarrhythmia was unlikely in view of the 2-week time course. Likewise, pulmonary embolus typically does not present over this time period (Tables 3.2 and 3.3).

References

1. Beckman HB, Frankel RM (1984) The effect of physician behavior on the collection of data. Ann Intern Med 101:692–696
2. Marvel MK, Epstein RM, Flowers K, Beckman HB (1999) Soliciting the patient' agenda: have we improved? JAMA 281:283–287
3. Osler W (1904) The master-word in medicine. In: Aequanimites with other addresses to medical students, nurses, and practitioners of medicine. Blakiston, Philadelphia, PA
4. Graber ML, Franklin N, Gordon R (2005) Diagnostic errors in internal medicine. Arch Intern Med 165:1493–1499
5. Morgan WL, Engel GL (1969) The clinical approach to the patient. WB Saunders, Philadelphia, PA
6. Kliegman RM (2004) Acute and chronic abdominal pain. In: Kliegman RM, Greenbaum LA, Lye PS (eds) Practical strategies in pediatric diagnosis and therapy, 2nd edn. Elsevior Saunders, Philadelphia, PA
7. Smith RC (2002) Patient-centered interviewing: an evidence-based method, 2nd edn. Lippincott Williams and Wilkens, Philadelphia, PA
8. Coulehan JC, Block MR (2006) The medical interview in mastering skills for clinical practice, 5th edn. F.A. Davis, Philadelphia, PA
9. Sackett DL, Haynes RB, Guyatt GN, Tugwell P (1991) Clinical epidemiology: a basic science for clinical medicine, 2nd edn. Little, Brown, Boston, MA
10. Barrows HS, Norman GR, Neufield VR, Feightner JW (1982) The clinical reasoning of randomly selected physicians in general medical practice. Clin Invest Med 5:49–55
11. Kuhn GJ (2002) Diagnostic errors. Acad Emerg Med 9:740–750
12. Platt FW, Gordon GH (2004) Field guide to the difficult interview, 2nd edn. Lippincott Williams and Wilkins, Philadelphia, PA
13. Roter DL, Hall JA (2006) Doctors talking with patients/patients talking with doctors: improving communication in medical visits, 2nd edn. Praeger, Westport, CT
14. University of Pittsburgh-Teaching Times (2006) November, vol XII
15. Chungs SS, Gerber P, Kirlin KA (2006) Ictal eye closure is a reliable indicator for psychogenic nonepileptic seizures. Neurology 66:1730–1731
16. Davis G, Henderson MC, Smetana GW (2005) The evidence-based approach to clinical decision making. In: Tierny LM, Henderson MC (eds) The patient history: evidence-based approach. Large Medical Book/McGraw Hill, New York

17. Sylvester FA, Hyams JS (2004) Gastrointestinal bleeding. In: Kliegman RM, Greenbaum LA, Lye PS (eds) Practical strategies in pediatric diagnosis and therapy, 2nd edn. Elsevier Saunders, Philadelphia, PA

18. Becker T, Kharhanda A, Bucher R (2007) Atypical clinical features of pediatric appendicitis. Acad Emerg Med 14:124–129

19. Platt FW, McMath JC (1979) Clinical hypocompetence: the interview. Ann Intern Med 91:898–902

20. Shea SC (1998) Psychiatric interviewing: the art of understanding: a practical guide for psychiatrists, psychologists, nurses, and other mental health pprofessionals, 2nd edn. WB Saunders, Philadelphia, PA

21. Korsch BM, Aley EF (1973) Pediatric interviewing techniques: current pediatric therapy. Sci Am 3:1–42

22. Mishler EG (1984) The discourse of medicine: dialectics of medical interviews. Ablex, Norwood, NJ

23. Gould RK, Rothenberg MB (1973) The chronically ill child facing death: how can the pediatrician help. Clin Pediatr 12:447–449

4

Concluding Phase

*We needed to understand seizures, to understand the effects of
the medications, but most of all we needed help to understand
all the things that were happening to our children and to us.*

> –Anonymous Parent, *Seizures and Epilepsy
> in Childhood: A Guide for Parents* by John
> Freeman, Eileen Vining, and Diana Pillas

Case: Jenny, a 2-year-old girl with a resolving pneumonia and pleu-
ral effusion, breathes comfortably on the toddler unit of the hospital. She recently transferred to the floor after an admission to
the pediatric intensive care unit. Her nurse reports to the first year
resident that Jenny's parents keep asking when Jenny can go home.
John, a first year resident, recalls how ill Jenny looked just 3 days
ago. Surprised at the parent's request, John walks down to Jenny's
room to talk with them.

Parents may make this type of inquiry as a way to reassure
themselves. "She must be okay if she is going home from the hospital." Some parents avoid asking specific questions about their
child's illness when frightened. John must avoid the temptation to
rush the discharge discussion of Jenny's illness with this family,
just because they seem in a rush to go home.

A clinician in the outpatient setting can also feel time pressure.
He might have spent excessive time on the data-gathering stage of
an interview and wants to hurry through the closing phase so that
he can move to the next patient. Alternatively, a clinician might
simply discount the importance of the closing. That is a mistake.
The success of the concluding phase largely determines the success
of implementing an effective treatment plan [1]. ***The importance***

J. Binder, *Pediatric Interviewing: A Practical, Relationship-Based
Approach*, Current Clinical Practice, DOI 10.1007/978-1-60761-256-8_4,
© Springer Science+Business Media, LLC 2010

of this phase should not be undermined by giving quick or premature responses to patients during earlier stages in the interview when they ask a question or express a self-diagnosis leading them to worry. Their question or worry can be acknowledged with the advisement that you will fully discuss the diagnosis and treatment options after your evaluation.

Clinician: I see you are worried that this might be a clot in her lungs or pneumonia. Lots of conditions can cause these symptoms, most of them not serious. I will talk to you about this as soon as I have all the information I need.

Comment: Sometimes, as in this case, the parents are worried about the same diagnosis as we are (pneumonia). We still can ask them to hold the worry until we get a bit more information. Later we can praise them for their diagnostic acumen and clarify by adding our own ideas.

An effective closing requires the following:

- Time – a prerequisite.
- A thorough knowledge of the diagnosis in question
- The ability to explain the condition and treatment in clear, straightforward language
- The ability to uncover fears and misperceptions
  The willingness to negotiate

Michael Rothenberg listed five basic questions that must be answered to accomplish the goals of this part of the interview. These questions provide the framework for the closing.

1. What do I have?
2. How did I get it?
3. Why did I get it?
4. What is going to be done about it?
5. What will my course be? [2]

The answer to these questions leads to a shared understanding of the child's condition. The shared understanding allows for a real partnership in implementing a treatment plan. The family assimilates accurate information only after any distortions they hold regarding the illness are resolved. This makes the closing part of the interview a give and take process; the family's understanding is checked each step of the way. This stage might be straightforward for a child with an ear or sinus infection, but the process remains a give and take discussion.

Let us take a look at the process for a family bringing a child for follow-up after a febrile seizure.

Case: Outpatient follow-up visit for 12-month-old Emily who was seen 2 days ago in the ER after a brief febrile seizure. Her development and neurological exam are normal. Parents report no family history of seizures. As the physician sits down to answer the five basic questions for Emily's mother, she notices that Mrs. Phillips' face is drawn and she appears stressed.

Physician:	It sounds like you have had a real stressful week. Let's talk about your understanding of Emily's condition.
Comment:	Obtaining the family's view of the illness provides the information needed to correct any misperceptions and develop a common understanding.
Mrs. Phillips:	The emergency room doctor diagnosed a febrile seizure. She shook all over. She turned blue. She was gurgling and making noises. It came out of nowhere. She seemed well when I put her down for a nap.
Comment:	Anything that seems to come out of nowhere is going to be mysterious and upsetting. No wonder Mrs. Phillips is stressed.
Physician:	It sounds frightening.
Mrs. Phillips:	Yes.
Physician:	What worried you the most?
Mrs. Phillips:	Her breathing. She wasn't breathing.
Physician:	Tell me about that.
Mrs. Phillips:	I didn't see her breathing. I didn't know what to do.
Physician:	Some parent's fear that their child is dying when they witness their child turning blue and having a seizure. It that true for you? (third person technique)
Mrs. Phillips:	I really thought she was dying.
Physician:	And what do you think about that now?
Mrs. Phillips:	I stay awake at night thinking of the possibility Emily might have a seizure and die.

Physician:	No wonder you feel stressed. Let's talk about febrile seizures. Just as people in society communicate with one another, the cells in the brain are connected to other cells in the brain. Cells send messages to one another using minute amounts of electricity. This is usually an orderly process. But problems in sending these messages can occur, just as they do in society. One factor that can make cells misfire in young children is fever [3]. Emily's fever triggered the seizure.
Mrs. Phillips:	Why did Emily develop a fever in the first place?
Physician:	We will come back to that as soon as we finish discussing her seizure. Is that okay?
Mrs. Phillips:	Yes.
Physician:	Earlier you said you were fearful of Emily having a seizure and dying.
Mrs. Phillips:	Yes.
Physician:	During Emily's seizure, her brain cells misfired. This caused her muscles to jerk, including the muscles controlling her breathing. She was breathing and getting oxygen. She was not dying. Her lips turned blue because the oxygen was going to more important organs than her skin—specifically her brain and heart. In a recent study of over 300 children who had a seizure and no brain conditions like a stroke, no child died during the five years of the study [4]. I feel confident in saying Emily's risk of dying is no different than a child without a history of febrile seizure. But, I know it can be terrifying to witness a seizure.
Mrs. Phillips:	It sure is.
Comment:	Emily's mother appears calmer once her fear has been addressed. The clinician will check her understanding before moving onto the next topic. Patients' recall and comprehension has been estimated to be as low as 50% [5]. This is especially likely for patients with low health literacy [5]. Clinicians can reduce this ineffective communication by asking the patient to *restate* what they heard the clinician say [5].

Physician: To make sure I have explained myself clearly, will you tell me what you heard me say about a benign seizure due to fever?

Mrs. Phillips: Well. A seizure occurs when the brain cells send too much electricity to other brain cells. This causes the muscles to jerk.

Physician: Right. And, what about the cause?

Comment: It is rare for a physician to close the loop—checking back with the patient to make sure the patient and doctor have a shared understanding. This may be due to a fear of taking too much time, even though studies show visits are no longer when patient understanding is checked [5].

Mrs. Phillips: Fever can do it, especially in young children.

Physician: Okay. What about your scare about what can happen during a benign febrile seizure like Emily experienced? Do you believe you need to stay awake and watch her sleep?

Mrs. Phillips: Not so much. But, I'm still a little worried.

Physician: Tell me more.

Mrs. Philips: I believe what you are saying. It is going to take me time to get used to it.

Physician: Of course.

Comment: Education is not a one time event. Families with a chronic condition need re-education throughout the course of the illness.

Physician: Let's go over several practical issues. She needs to be watched when she bathes or goes swimming because of the risk of drowning.

Mrs. Phillips: I understand

Physician: If she would have another seizure, place her on her side and do not put anything in her mouth. "She will not swallow her tongue" [3]. Most febrile seizures stop within a couple of minutes. If it lasts longer than five minutes or recurs, you will need to call an ambulance.

Mrs. Phillips: Okay

Physician:	Do you have other concerns about Emily's seizure. Some parents have concerns about possible brain damage or even mental retardation [6]. (third person technique).
Mrs. Phillips:	No, I know she is a smart girl.
Physician:	Earlier you asked about the cause of Emily's fever. (Referred gate)
Mrs. Phillips:	Why did she have a fever?
Physician:	She had a viral infection in her throat causing the fever. The physician in the emergency room examined Emily to make sure her fever was not due to an infection of the brain or it's covering. I agree.
Mrs. Phillips:	Okay. What can I do now about preventing another seizure?
Physician:	We can prevent most febrile seizures if we prescribe a daily medication. I don't recommend that for several reasons. We estimate that Emily has a 70% chance she will not experience another febrile seizure [3]. Another febrile seizure would not damage her brain, cause mental retardation or death as we have already discussed. Medications have the risk of significant side effects-including behavioral problems like being hyperactive. I would not recommend medicine.
Mrs. Phillips:	I understand. I didn't want to put Emily on medication.
Physician:	Do you have any more questions?
Mrs. Phillips:	Will she have epilepsy when she grows up?
Physician:	Her chance of developing epilepsy is about the same as the chance of children who have never experienced a febrile seizure—97% chance she will not develop epilepsy. The medications we just discussed don't decrease that risk [3]. Before we finish I would like to make a recommendation.
Mrs. Phillips:	Please tell me.
Physician:	Set clear limits on her behavior like you would for any child. A temper tantrum because she hears "no" does not cause seizures. Here is a pamphlet

on febrile seizures to take home and read. Please call me if you have any questions.

Comment: An effective closing takes time so that he five basic questions can be asked and answered. When the clinician structures the interview so that he gives himself time for each phase of the interview, he can smoothly accomplish his goals for the overall encounter.

References

1. Shea SC (1998) Psychiatric interviewing: the art of understanding: a practical guide for psychiatrics, psychologists, nurses, and other mental health professional, 2nd edn. W.B. Saunders, Philadelphia, PA
2. Rothenberg MB (1974) The unholy trinity: activity, authority, and magic. Clin Pediatr 13:870–873
3. Freeman JM, Vining EPG, Pillas DJ (2002) Seizures and epilepsy in childhood: a guide for parents, 3rd edn. The John Hopkins University Press, Baltimore, MD
4. Cullenbach MC, Westendorp GJ, Geerts AT et al (2001) Mortality risk in children with epilepsy: the Dutch study of epilepsy in childhood. Pediatrics 107:1259–1263
5. Schillinger D, Piette J, Grumbach K et al (2003) Closing the loop: physician communication with diabetic patients who have low health literacy. Arch Intern Med 163:83–90
6. Mittan RJ (2005) Seizures and epilepsy education program parent's manual: how to raise a child with epilepsy, part 1: coping with fear. EP Mag October:60–66. http://www.eparent.com

5
Family

Something in our nature cries out to be loved by another. Isolation is devastating to the human psyche. That is why solitary confinement is considered to be the cruelest of punishments.

Gary Chapman, *The Five Languages of Love*

Less than 50 years ago since Wynne and Singer published a study connecting poor outcome in schizophrenia with living in a family marred by hostility and conflict [1]. Today, research has established that patients with diabetes, asthma, and other *physical* conditions do worse in the context of a critical or harsh family environment [2]. Critical and rejecting environments lead to poorer outcomes: nurturing environments improve the health of family members. Families can help clarify a problem or situation, encourage lifestyle changes, promote adherence to treatment recommendations, and even impact the actual physiology of a medical condition [3].

Case: Jeremy is a thin, bespectacled, 14-year-old, eighth grader with dyslexia and a history of diabetes mellitus for 11 years. Henry and his mother had smoothly controlled the diabetes mellitus until six months ago. He has been hospitalized twice for diabetic ketoacidosis (dka) in the last three months. His grades, previously B's, have slipped to C's and D's. He frequently argues with his mother over monitoring of his blood glucose levels and the timing of his insulin injections. Jeremy lived with his 38-year-old mother Janet and his 12-year-old sister Andrea. He visits his biological father infrequently. His parents divorced nine years ago. During the second hospitalization, Jeremy's pediatrician convenes a family conference.

J. Binder, *Pediatric Interviewing: A Practical, Relationship-Based Approach,* Current Clinical Practice, DOI 10.1007/978-1-60761-256-8_5, © Springer Science+Business Media, LLC 2010

The task for Jeremy's pediatrician is to harness the power in these family relationships and help move them in a positive direction in order to change the course of Henry's diabetes. In this chapter, I describe the benefits of a family approach for a child with a chronic condition like diabetes, as well as for any child presenting to the pediatrician for care. This chapter will:

- Define family and discuss several ideas central to understanding family. The concepts will provide a common basis of meaning.
- Describe strategies for obtaining information about family relationships and family dynamics (SOCIAL HISTORY).
- Discuss three variations of a family visit.
- Explore the use of a family conference with a family having a child with a chronic condition.

FAMILIES

Fewer than 50% of families now consist of the traditional two parent families [4]. Most children live in single-parent families, grandparent-led families, same sex parent families, or blended families. Any definition of family must take this into account. As I was wrestling with this task of defining family, I was reminded of a comment made by a father of a 4-year-old boy named Angel, a patient of mine during my residency in New York City 30 years ago. Angel's mother was concerned about his lack of minding at home. When I asked the father about his view of the situation he responded:

"It's not my fault. I'm never home."

I was struck by the irony of this remark. As I think back at that remark, I have questions:

- Did this father believe he was not an important member of the family because he worked long hours away from home? If so, how could he be invited to participate in Angel's health care?
- Did he believe the healthcare profession was looking to find problems and place blame on the family? If so, how could he be helped to alter this view?
- What was this man's experience of family growing up? How did that influence his current relationships?

Carter and McGoldrick emphasize that the emotional life of a family includes three or four generations of people. Members of one household react to past, present, and even anticipated future relationships within that family system [5]. Kadis and McCelndin define family *"to be a group of people who have a kinship bond and currently share a common experience* [6]." They use the metaphor of a car engine to help the reader visualize each family as a system. Just as the individual parts (cylinders, pistons, etc.) of a car engine laid out end-to-end on a garage floor do not make an engine, so too with the individual members of a family [6]. In any system, such as a family, one part influences and is influenced by other parts. For example, a wife may believe her husband does not spend enough time with their children and anxiously tells him to spend more time with them. Only, the husband perceives this as hassling. He responds by pouting and spending less time with the children, which increases his wife's anxiety and reminders. If either of them would change their response, the negative cycle could be broken. If the wife remained warm and playful, the husband would be more likely to become engaged with the children; if the husband stopped pouting and became curious about his wife's anxiety, she probably would calm down [7].

Typically outside of their awareness, parents repeat the patterns of interaction between family members they saw modeled growing up, some helpful, others not [8]. These patterns can be changed by life events such as divorce, chronic illness, early parental death, or by a family's intentional effort to change. In addition to understanding these intergeneration patterns, a family-focused clinician considers four other dimensions of family: level of functioning; family life cycle; family structure; and family process [8]. Understanding a family along those four dimensions enhances the clinician's ability to join and help the family.

Level of Functioning
Stephen Shultz described four levels of family functioning – psychotic, immature, neurotic, and mature. The family at the immature level does not talk out feelings or needs or resolve problems. Instead, one of the members acts out through substance abuse, an eating disorder, a personality disorder, or physical or sexual abuse. The neurotic family has a member who uses ineffective coping strategies, leading to anxiety or depression. For example, a 12-year-old boy is diagnosed with social anxiety in the context of critical parenting. Families at the mature level talk out their needs and feelings and solve problems [8, 9]. Many pediatricians consider counseling families with problems at the psychotic or immature level to be outside their level of expertise.

Family Life Cycle

Families with children progress through predictable stages. Young adults leave home, form a couple relationship, bear children, and raise them. During each stage of the life cycle, families face specific developmental tasks, which repeat when their children have children. Families need to pull together during the child bearing years, a centripetal period; while they must become more open to the extrafamilial environment during adolescence, a centrifugal period [10].

> "When illness occurs during a centripetal period, like infancy, the family may be more easily mobilized to care for the ill member then it is during a centrifugal period like adolescence when the individual, is moving toward increased independence from one another. Parents of teenagers with diabetes, for example, are notorious for having difficulty helping their children balance their need for autonomy with the demands of the illness" [3].

The individual's movement through his or her own life cycle takes place within the context of the family life cycle. Parents with young children must balance starting their career and developing a healthy couple relationship with the constant time constraints involved in caring for young children. A parent raising teenage children will typically have fewer physical demands, but may be coping with the multiple losses that come with middle age or be dealing with the demands involved in caretaking an elderly parent [5].

Family Structure

Another key dimension for describing families is the distribution of power and authority in the family:

Are the parents in charge?

Are the boundaries between parent and child clear and appropriate?

Is the structure flexible enough to allow access of one individual with everyone else?

Are there alliances (or coalitions) among members?

How does the family deal with emotional closeness and distance? [3, p. 36]

A common structural issue in alcoholic families is a reversal of roles [11]. An older child takes on parental responsibilities (e.g., supervising younger children neglected by the parents). This child helps solve a family problem at a cost of giving up a large part of her childhood. It is a big loss.

Family Process
Interpersonal processes can be analyzed by assessing family members using the following parameters.

Differentiation
Differentiation refers to the process of a child (or adult) growing in her ability to think her own thoughts, feel her own feelings, and take action to get her own needs met. To the extent differentiation is not supported by a family, a tendency will exist for a child to get "triangulated" in the parental system. Parents triangulate a child when they diffuse their tension with each other by both focusing their energy on the child [8]. Triangulated children can develop a myriad of symptoms, from anxiety to eating disorders.

Basic Belief About Okayness
Okayness has to do with an individual's belief about her own essential nature and is the driving force underlying her behavior and life experience [8]. Children who believe their essence is okay act in positive ways; children who believe they are not okay exhibit negative behaviors.

"Stroking" Pattern
In Transactional Analysis terminology, a stroke is "any act implying recognition of another's presence" [12]. The type (positive or negative; conditional or unconditional) and frequency are noted. A paucity of stokes or an increased ratio of negative strokes might be present in a depressed family. Often parents inadvertently reinforce negative behavior by stroking it. For example, a parent makes a comment every time a child makes a mistake and ignores positive behavior.

> "Changing the stroking pattern allows the members to reinforce a different kind of behavior. Until the stroking pattern is changed, it is difficult for individuals in the family to change because they are being reinforced for their typical behaviors." [8] Vann Joines

Family Mood
Many families have a prevailing mood such as depression, anxiety, or frustration that has been reinforced time and again within the family [8]. If the prevailing mood is frustration, it is likely members respond to an individual's frustration, but not when the member is sad or happy.

SOCIAL HISTORY

It is common for clinicians to express anxiety when faced with doing a family interview. Physicians in training are expected to know how to obtain a social history, often without any real training, since it has been a low educational priority. It is no wonder that students present abbreviated social histories:

> "Jeremy has two parents, who are divorced, and a younger sister. He is in 8th grade. They have city water."

The following interviewing approaches and techniques will provide the clinician with the tools needed to create a safe, supportive environment for the family and allow the clinician to gather an adequate family database. An adequate family database must include information about the dynamics and quality of the family relationships:

1. One may begin by joining with the family. The tools used to engage with an individual, discussed in Chap. 2, are useful in joining with a family.

   - Greet each member, no matter the age.
   - Adopt an unconditional positive regard for each family member. Affirm the strengths of the family.
   - Ask questions of and show interest in each person while identifying demographic data and special interests or talents of the individuals. Track with the family conversation:

     > "Since I haven't met you before, tell me a little about yourself. Tell me what you see as your family's biggest strength. What do you do in the way of fun activities?"

   - Establish an agreement or *contract* for the meeting.

Clinician:	You and I have not discussed your wife's concerns about Jeremy. Did you want to come to today's family conference?
Mr. Garber:	Not really.
Clinician:	How did you decide to come, then?
Mr. Garber:	I don't think Jeremy has a problem, but I wanted to support my wife.
Clinician:	Given that is how you made your decision to participate, is there anything you would want to get out of today's meeting?

- Elicit and validate family members' feelings. It is often helpful to identify underlying feelings when a family member is reactive or expressing disagreement. A common underlying emotion in that situation is anxiety.

2. Use open-ended questions, particularly gentle commands to obtain each person's views about the situation or relationship.

   "Tell me how you feel about your relationship with your spouse."
   "Describe what your relationship with your son Jeremy is like."

3. Incorporate Behavioral Incidents. This technique is discussed in Chap. 8 as a validity technique. It is an easy-to-use tool for uncovering specific information about relationships [13]. The tone and other characteristics of the parent–child relationship are revealed as the clinician asks for concrete details of a recent interaction in the family.

   A parent is asked to describe a recent day in the life of a child. The parent provides specific data about the child getting up in the morning, getting dressed, eating, interacting, playing, watching TV, communicating, reacting to limits.

   Or

   A parent is asked to pick an example of a problematic behavior from the last 1–2 weeks. They then describe the parental and child interactions in detail.

   "He hit his little sister on the top of her head. I went over and asked why he did that. He said he didn't know. I then...."

   At the conclusion of the incident the parent is asked what she is feeling, what she is thinking about the child, and what she is saying to herself about herself as a parent or person. A corollary of this technique is to have the parent put themselves back in the situation and describe it as if it were happening now. This may give the parent better access to the feelings they experienced at the time of the incident.

   "Describe the situation in the first person present tense, as if it were occurring right now. Just let yourself be there."

4. Use Circular Questioning. Circular questioning is a style of interviewing developed by the Milan Associates (Selvini et al.). The purpose of circular questioning is to obtain information about the **_differences or changes_** in the relationships in the family that have occurred as a result of the problem [14]. It is a clever and powerful tool. Once learned, it is easy to use and provides good information about relationship dynamics.

Sarah is describing how her 8-year-old son would not do his homework when she tells him to do it. She describes becoming frustrated and giving up. The interviewer turns to the father and asks him what he experiences when his wife is telling her son to do his homework and his son does not comply.

"What do you feel when you listen to their interaction?"

"What do you think about their interaction?"

The information that the father provides helps the interviewer set up the next question. For example, if the father says he thinks she is too harsh and he withdraws, the interviewer may then ask the mother:

"So, when your husband withdraws as your son resists doing his homework, what's that like for you?"

"What do you feel?

What do you do as a result?"

In the above example, the interviewer obtains information about how well the parents work together without asking directly. Directly asking about the quality of a relationship is another option, but can lead to defensiveness in some families.

5. Set up an enactment. The information is right in front of the physician with this method. Two people in the family are asked to talk to each other about a situation [15]. The interaction occurs live in the office. Family therapists often make use of this tool. There is no reason pediatricians cannot take advantage of this uniquely helpful technique, as long as they set up the enactment so that the participants face each other and are encouraged to talk and listen to each other regarding a specific topic and for a specified time period. John and Linda are parents who have just described their different approaches to their 15-year-old son, who has been smoking marijuana regularly. The physician asks them:

Physician: Would you be willing to talk with each other about the problem? It seems you have different ideas about how to help your son. Talk to each other as if I am not here.

Parents: We have already done that at home.

Physician: Would you do it anyway?

Parents: Okay.

Bader and Pierson suggest watching each partner's ability to: stick to one topic, express his/her thinking *and* feelings on the subject, and to do so without attacking the other. The clinician also observes each partner's ability to listen carefully and express empathy for their partner [16].

6. Take a relationship history as a part of the developmental history. The interviewer starts with the pregnancy and asks about the character of the parent–child interactions at each stage of development. Questions about the parental system can be woven into the conversation (e.g., How did parents decide what was most important in raising their children? How do they spend their leisure time? How do they resolve their differences?)

7. Make use of normalization techniques such as the third person technique. Family members unaccustomed to talking out issues as a family can feel uncomfortable and vulnerable. Normalization eases their anxiety.

> "Jeremy, lots of kids who have diabetes feel resentful and believe that it's not fair that the other kids in the family don't have to check their blood sugars. Is that true for you?"

8. Pay attention to nonverbal communication. As we noted in Chap. 2, people reveal themselves more nonverbally than verbally, mostly out of their own awareness. It is helpful for the clinician to assess the nonverbal behavior of family members. Who sits close to whom? What is their body posture like? Is there eye contact with each other? What are they revealing by their tone or pace of speech?

> Colleen is twelve years old and experiencing social anxiety. She appears shy and cuddles up next to mom on the couch. Dad takes a seat across the room from mom. The clinician forms a hypothesis regarding family dynamics: she considers the possibility of mom being overly involved with Colleen and dad being more distant.

This list of interviewing techniques useful for taking a social history is not all-inclusive. It does have enough variety to meet the needs of a primary care clinician taking a social history. The bottom line is that a good family or social history must include data about relationships, since families, by definition, are relational.

VARIATIONS OF FAMILY VISIT

A pediatrician committed to a family-oriented approach must *"think family."* Thomas Campbell and his collaborators described *thinking family* with individual patients as one of the three ways a clinician can be involved with a family [17]. Thinking family means asking family-oriented questions, such as:

"Has anyone else in the family had this problem?"

"What do family members believe caused the problem and how should it be treated?"

"Who in the family is most concerned about the problem?"

"Along with your illness, have there been any other recent changes or stresses in your life?"

"How can your family or friends be helpful to you in dealing with this problem?" [3]

The key concept is that the individual's illness affects his family and at the same time is affected by his family. Pediatricians must *think family* when older adolescents make individual appointments. The routine pediatric visit with parents and child attending the visit defines the second type of family involvement. Strategies for interviewing during this type of visit are identical to the recommendations for conducting a family conference, the third form of a family visit. The *family conference* is a specially arranged meeting by either the physician or the family to discuss a health or family problem in more detail. Families readily accept family conferences [3].

Family Conference

The family-oriented pediatrician convenes a family conference as a routine aspect of pediatrics, just as she would order liver function tests if indicated. Indications include serious family problems or conflicts, hospitalizations, giving bad news, or simply recommending lifestyle changes [3]. In the case of Jeremy, he has been hospitalized twice in 3 months. Before the actual meeting Dr. Elisa reviews Jeremy's chart and formulates specific goals for the meeting, as well as a tentative hypothesis about the family situation.

- Dr. Elisa's goal is to explore relationship dynamics and inquire about their impact on Jeremy's diabetes.
- Jeremy is moving into the stage of increasing psychological independence. Mrs. Ayers, a single mother works to support the family. The family is moving from the stage of raising young children to the stage of promoting independence in their adolescent children.
- Dr. Elisa's hypotheses is that Mrs. Ayers is having difficulty making the transition to supporting increasing independence in the children and this is negatively impacting the diabetes.
- Dr. Elisa contacts Mrs. Ayers and discusses her reason for proposing the meeting: develop a better understanding of what is

contributing to Jeremy's poorly controlled diabetes in order to resolve the problem. She gets an agreement that Mrs. Ayers, Jeremy, and his sister Andrea will attend. It is important that the family understand all members are expected to attend (the only contraindication to this is the potential of violence after such a meeting – history of domestic violence) [3]. The family needs to know what will be discussed, so that there are no surprises or sabotaging of the meeting.

- Dr. Elisa will structure the family conference using the three-phase interviewing structure she utilizes in any interview with opening, middle, and closing phases.

Opening Phase
The clinician has several tasks during this phase:

- Introduce herself, greet each member of the family, and get to know each member. She will *join* with the family using standard engagement strategies.
- Elicit each member's goal for the session in concrete, behavioral terms. The clinician can also propose any goals that she believes are important. Prioritize the goals.

Dr. Elisa: Okay, Mrs. Ayers, now that we have heard your hopes for the session, let's move to Jeremy. Jeremy, tell me what you would like to be better.

Jeremy: I want mom to get off my back about checking my blood sugar levels and taking my insulin.

Mrs. Ayers (interrupting): I would get off your back if you were responsible.

Jeremy (interrupting): You never give me a chance to be responsible.

Dr. Elisa: Lets take this part one person at a time. Jeremy, it sounds like your goal is to be more in charge of managing your diabetes. Is that right?

Comment: One important rule for healthy family functioning is to have each person speak his own thoughts and feelings. This is called differentiation. The Ayers family is struggling with the issue of differentiation. Based on his history with the Ayers, Dr. Elisa mentally places them along the other family dimensions described earlier in the chapter:

Level of functioning – *Symptoms suggest neurotic level.*

Family life cycle – They are in the stage of promoting independence (adolescent) and will soon be approaching the launching phase.

Structure – Mrs. Ayer takes a parental role and establishes clear boundaries.

Process – The individuals in the family appear undifferentiated. Mrs. Ayers's use of negative strokes has increased emotional distance. Jeremy responds from a "not okay" position and acts irresponsibly. The family mood is anxious.

Middle Phase

The tasks of this middle phase include:

- Elicit each person's view of the problem. Gentle commands, behavioral incidents, enactments, and circular questioning are helpful tools with this task. The clinician provides leadership by not allowing one member to monopolize the conversation; not allowing members to interrupt each other; and not taking sides.
- Identify strengths in the family. A family member might have a big heart but have difficulty verbalizing her caring.
- Discern what the bottom line issue is for the family, if enough information is obtained [8].

Dr. Elisa:	Andrea, tell me what you think is the main problem.
Andrea:	Jeremy takes up all of mom's time, because he doesn't do what he is supposed to do.
Dr. Elisa:	What's that like for you?
Andrea:	I don't like it. It's not fair.
Dr. Elisa:	It sounds like you and Jeremy have that in common. Neither of you think it is fair. You think Jeremy gets too much attention. Jeremy believes it is unfair that he is the one who has to check his blood sugars, watch his diet and take insulin.
Andrea:	I guess that's true.
Dr. Elisa:	Andrea, would you be willing to do an experiment. Would you talk to mom about this? You know, how you think Jeremy takes up your mom's energy and there is not enough left for you.
Andrea:	Okay

Mrs. Ayers:	Andrea, I sort of know you felt this way all along.
Andrea:	Then, how come you do it?
Mrs. Ayers:	Jeremy has diabetes. It's not easy for him to have to check his blood sugars all the time and take insulin.
Andrea: Jeremy.	I know. It's just that everything seems to be about
Mrs. Ayers:	I worry about him.
Dr. Elisa:	Mrs. Ayers, what is your biggest worry?
Mrs. Ayers:	I worry that his diabetes will get out of control.... That he could die.
Dr. Elisa:	What a big worry!
Mrs. Ayers:	Yes it's huge, especially since Jeremy doesn't monitor his blood sugars like he is supposed to unless I remind him.
Jeremy:	You never give me a chance. You're always telling me to watch my diet, check my blood sugars. I never get a break.
Comment:	It is important for a family with a chronic condition to verbalize underlying feelings of anxiety, resentment, anger, guilt, sadness in a safe or supportive manner. When feelings are expressed and talked about they can be resolved. Otherwise, they can fester and poison the family interactions. The pattern of interactions demonstrated by the Ayers family easily becomes entrenched. The parent hovers and the teen rebels. The more the parent hovers, the more the teen rebels. With diabetes mellitus, the rebellion can lead to death. Foster Cline and Lisa Greene recommend a "Love and Logic" approach for families that have previously emphasized love, concern, and giving lots and lots of suggestions (This approach is recommended only for those types of families). They suggest the parent show empathy and support for the child but allow the child to make choices and manage his or her own life:

"When you were a child, we treated you as a child, giving guidance, helping you make decisions, and sometimes telling you what to do and how to handle things. Parents do that for little kids. Now you are a teen and you think like a teen. God has provided you with some things that can either crack you or build your character, that can either lead to an increased awareness of life and its beauty or to unhappy decisions that will lead to death. We are both interested and curious about which path you will take" [18].

Concluding Phase

Like the concluding phase of any interview, the concluding phase of a family conference is done in a give-and-take format. The family's understanding and opinions are checked along the way. The tasks are:

- Educate family regarding the chronic illness and how it impacts the family's movement through the life cycle.
- Find a common theme that can help solve the problem. State it in a positive way.
- Ask for a commitment from each family member to a plan of action. ("Let's meet weekly for three weeks.")

Dr. Elisa: Do you have any concerns about the plan.

Mrs. Ayers: No.

Jeremy &
Andrea: No.

Dr. Elisa: Okay. It sounds like the main issue is that you all care for each other very much. In fact, so much that you tend to overdo and try to make things Okay for the other person, instead of asking the other person what they are feeling or wanting. The tendency is to jump in to help. This causes the other person to get upset since as a family, the children are in the stage of developing increasing independence. Sadly, Jeremy responds by not taking good care of his diabetes. Your agreement today is to stop and talk with the other person about the situation before jumping in to help. We practiced a new way of talking things out today. You agreed to experiment with this over the next week? We will meet in one week. Is that okay?

Everybody: Okay.

During the next three sessions Dr. Elisa will help this family cope with a ***chronic illness***. Because of her knowledge of pediatrics, as well as her understanding of common effects of a chronic condition on a family, she is ideally suited to help this family talk out and normalize feelings, including "unacceptable feelings" [19]. She will work to increase the children's and family's sense of self-efficacy and control by providing sound information about the condition and supporting family members making choices about what they can control [3]. Love and Logic parenting principles can be used to help families develop this type of resilience [18].

Primary care physicians must educate *and* reeducate families with chronic conditions. In the process, they can help parents balance the needs of the child who is ill with the needs of the other children and encourage family members to stay connected with others outside the family, since the demands of the illness can get in the way of connection with others [3].

Before closing this chapter, one further issue needs to be addressed. Many pediatricians, whether due to lack of adequate training or due to comfort level, may not be able or may not choose to do this level of family work. Rather, they may choose to affiliate with a mental health professional. The bottom line is that good pediatric care includes family in the assessment and treatment of children – both well and sick children. For the pediatrician who maintains a family-oriented approach, one of the best resources is developing an ongoing relationship with a certified family therapist. Helpful textbook resources include:

- *Family-Focused Behavioral Pediatrics* by William Lord Coleman (2001)
- *Family-Oriented Primary Care* (2nd ed.) by Susan McDaniel, Thomas L. Campbell, Jeri Hepworth, and Alan Lorenz (2005)
- *Parenting Children with Health Issues* by Foster Cline and Lisa Greene (2007) (Table 5.1)

TABLE 5.1. Family-oriented conference

Evaluation
Contact each family member
Contract with each individual
Check out each individual's perception of the problem
Use effective tools to obtain a social history
Management
Organize the data
What is the bottom line issue?
Present bottom line issue positively.
Ask for a commitment to a plan of action

References

1. Wynne LC, Singer MT (1963) Pseudo-mutuality in the family relations of schizophrenics. Arch Gen Psychiatry 9:11–200
2. Campbell TL, Patterson JM (1995) The effectiveness of family interventions in the treatment of physical illness. J Marital Fam Ther 21:545–583
3. McDaniel SH, Campbell TL, Hepworth J, Lorenz A (2005) Family-oriented primary care, 2nd edn. Springer, New York
4. US Bureau of the Census (2002) Statistical abstract of the United States: 2002, 121st edn. Current Population Survey, March 2002. US Bureau of the Census, Washington (DC)
5. Carter B, McGoldrick M (1989) Overview: the changing family cycle – a framework for family therapy. In: Carter B, McGoldrick M (eds) The changing family life cycle, 2nd edn. Allyn and Bacon, Boston, MA
6. Kadis LB, McClendon R (1998) Marital and family therapy. American Psychiatric Press, Washington, DC
7. Joines V (1985) Couples therapy. In: Kadis L (ed) Redecision therapy: expanded perspectives. Western Institute for Group and Family Therapy, Watsonville, CA
8. Joines V (2004) Redecision family therapy. In: Kalson FW (ed) Comprehensive handbook of psychotherapy, vol 3. Wiley, Hoboken, NJ
9. Shultz SJ (1984) Family system therapy and integration. Jason Aronson, New York
10. Combrinck-Graham LA (1985) Developmental model for family systems. Fam Proc 24:139–150
11. Black C (1987) It will never happen to me. Random House, New York
12. Berne E (1964) Games people play. Grove Press, New York
13. Pascal G (1983) The practical art of diagnostic interviews. Dow Jones-Irwin, Homewood, IL
14. Penn P (1982) Circular questioning. Fam Proc 21:267–280
15. Minuchin S, Fishman HC (1981) Family therapy techniques. Harvard University Press, Cambridge, MA
16. Bader E, Pearson PT (1988) In quest of the mythical mate: a developmental approach to diagnosis and treatment in couples therapy. Brunner/Mazel, New York
17. Cole-Kelly K., Seaburn D (1999) Five Areas of questioning to promote a family-oriented approach in primary care. Fam Syst Health 17:340–348
18. Cline FW, Greene LC (2007) Parenting children with health issues. Love and Logic Press, Golden, CO
19. McCollum A (1975) Coping with prolonged health impairment in your child. Little, Brown, Boston, MA

6
The Well-Child Visit

Child health care should be fun.......Through setting the agenda for each visit, setting up an office with a developmental focus and really connecting with families without hiding behind forms and checklists, the clinician can claim back some of the excitement of pediatric practice.

Suzanne D. Dixon and Martin T. Stein,
Encounters with Children, 4th ed:

Jack, a second year pediatric resident in continuity clinic, enters the exam room to see his first patient, Braxton, a six-year-old boy in kindergarten. Braxton performs poorly in school and has been suspended twice for spitting and fighting. He is markedly overweight. He spends his spare time watching TV and playing video games. Grandma watches him after school. Sadly, he reports no friends to play with in his neighborhood. Jack feels discouraged. He says to himself that he does not like well-child care and wants to go into neonatology.

Residents frequently take care of children living in poor families. Poor children often present with multiple health needs; poor families make do with sparse resources [1]. Although many residents look forward to caring for their own panel of patients in a continuity clinic, they often feel overwhelmed by the challenges their patients and families face. Even more problematic, many residents lack a clear, conceptual framework for structuring well-child care visits [2], most likely a direct result of two phenomena:

- The existence of an overwhelming number of recommendations for anticipatory guidance from governing organizations like the American Academy of Pediatrics and the Bright Futures Project.

J. Binder, *Pediatric Interviewing: A Practical, Relationship-Based Approach*, Current Clinical Practice, DOI 10.1007/978-1-60761-256-8_6, © Springer Science+Business Media, LLC 2010

• A lack of training in evidence-based strategies for helping families make lifestyle changes [2–4].

In my experience, this can lead to the use of checklists, poor rapport, and a lack of satisfaction for both parties involved. This chapter outlines a structure for well-child visits based on accepted principles of child and family development. A discussion of the purposes of well-child care will allow us to formulate a clear, effective game plan – one that supports that resident in continuity clinic. Well-child care in USA has most often been visualized as having two main tasks (1) screen for a host of developmental and medical conditions that might benefit from early treatment or referral and (2) provide anticipatory guidance and support.

Fifteen to eighteen percent of all children live with a developmental, behavioral, or emotional disorder [5]. Many children with devel opmental disorders exhibit subtle findings. The majority of these problems are missed at routine medical visits if only surveillance (physician observation) is used [5]. Identification and participation of children in early intervention programs leads to increased graduation from high school, avoidance of teenage delinquency, and independent living as adults [5, 6]. That is why the American Academy of Pediatrics recommends that formal developmental screens be used at well-child visits [7].

The amount of time developmental screening tests take to administer in pediatric practice presents a major impediment to their routine use. In addition, a number of screens lack adequate reliability and validity. Glascoe and Shapiro state that screening tests should have 70–80% reliability and validity so that almost all children with developmental problems will be identified if the tests are used longitudinally (9-, 18-, 30-month visits). Some practitioners accomplish this task by having parents complete a brief, reliable, and valid developmental questionnaire (e.g., Ages and Stages, PEDS) before the well-child visit [5]. Similarly, mental health conditions can be identified with the use of a comprehensive screen like the Pediatric Symptom Checklist (PSC or the PSC-17), given at acute care and health maintenance visits. These screens take approximately 5 min to be filled out.

This medical model is built on a strategy of screening for outliers. Sweden prefers to place their resources into promoting the positive development of all children with a family-centered, team approach, rather than routinely screen all children to identify problems [8].

ANTICIPATORY GUIDANCE

The second task of well-child care, anticipatory guidance, has been defined as the "provision of information to parents and children with the expected outcome being a change in parenting attitude or behavior [9]." Knowing a child's developmental strengths and weaknesses (task #1) allows the clinician to be responsive to a particular child and family.

Moyer and Butler, reporting on the scientific basis of well-child care, noted that common well-child interventions, such as counseling on nutrition, physical activity, and poison prevention, lack the support of a body of evidence demonstrating effectiveness [3]. When evidence is nonexistent or insufficient, physicians must rely on the experience and recommendation of experts. So, what do the experts say about anticipatory guidance and behavioral counseling?

The American Academy of Pediatrics, the Bright Futures Project, and the US Preventive Services Task Force list topics for routine behavioral counseling. These topics include safety/injury prevention; violence; guns; nutrition; sleep; exercise; play; nurturing and affirmations; family relationships; discipline; reading; TV; video games; sexual behavior; pregnancy prevention; smoking; passive smoke exposure; alcohol and drug use; and family adaptation to stress [10]. We face a problem with capacity. All the pediatricians in USA working round the clock could not cover these topics.

Trying to cover all the topics listed would be based on a flawed assumption regarding the process of how patients make behavioral or lifestyle changes. Patients do not change when they are given a talk or told what to do [11]. Let me illustrate this point: experts commonly suggest that clinicians talk to new parents about their adjustment as a family. We know 67% of new parents will become unhappy with their marital relationship in the next 3 years [12]. This negatively impacts the baby's emotional and cognitive development [12]. John Gottman, a world renowned expert on marriages, gave evening talks to educate couples regarding this phenomenon. These talks did not improve couple relationships [12]. If this world expert in couple dynamics could not change couple interaction patterns with a talk, it will not occur as a result a brief pediatric talk at the end of a well-child care visit.

Well-child visits often involve an invitation for the family to make a change: offer nutritious food, encourage exercise, do not smoke, read to your child, and limit television. The Gottman experience makes it clear that simply providing families with information is insufficient to promote change.

MOTIVATIONAL INTERVIEWING

To gain insight into the principles underlying lifestyle changes, we can look to the field of addiction. People with addictions to food, to drugs, to gambling... have long been considered to be resistant to change. Addicts were confronted with their denial. Change was seen as external to patients, something to be imposed on them for their own good [13].

In the late 1980s, counselors began having success with a different philosophical approach. They conceptualized change as a process residing within the patient. The counselor helped the patient identify and resolve his own ambivalence. Miller and Rollnick coined the term *motivational interviewing* to describe the counseling approach they created. Motivational interviewing elicits change with a directive, client-centered counseling style [13].

Using counseling principles congruent with virtually all schools of counseling and psychotherapy, Miller and Rollnick created motivational interviewing specifically to enhance the process of change. This makes it particularly well suited for promoting lifestyle or behavioral changes with families. Miller and Rollnick outline four general principles: express empathy; develop discrepancy; roll with resistance; and support self-efficacy [14]. Empathy includes seeing the patient's ambivalence as a normal part of the change process. "Acceptance facilitates change" [14]. The counselor attempts to illuminate the discrepancy between the patient's behavior and that patient's own personal goals or values. The counselor accepts the patient and her ambivalence, not the bad health behavior. He amplifies the discrepancy in order to invite the patient to make a behavioral change. He helps the patient identify important personal goals that are being affected by the behavior. When the counselor meets resistance, he simply takes that as a clue to move in a different direction. He does not debate with the patient. But the counselor may make an empathic summary statement to the patient: "It sounds like this topic isn't one you are eager to get into right now." Or, "It sounds like you have a lot of disagreements with this suggestion. I can imagine how it would not sit so well with you right now. Maybe we can address it another time." Questions are stated in a form that gives the problem back to the patient, so she finds her own solution. The counselor supports the patient's belief that she can indeed make the change. People do not attempt to change when they believe they are not capable of making the change. The counselor's belief in the patient's ability to change can be a powerful stimulus to the patient.

Keller and Kemp-White suggest asking the patient the two basic questions. A clinician first appraises the patient's motivation to change by asking about her belief in the value of change:

"How convinced are you that this behavior change is important to you? [15]"

She is asked to rate her conviction on a scale of 1–10, with 10 meaning her life is dependent on the change. The clinician can ask for clarification of her thinking;

"What would it take for your conviction to be a 7 instead of 3?"

Then, they suggest that the clinician appraise the patient's confidence in making such a change with a similar 1–10 scale.

"How confident are you that you can make that change? [15]"

This information helps the clinician plan treatment.

"A patient who is unconvinced may need to see data. A convinced but unconfident patient may need help planning simple steps toward change" [16]. (Platt and Gordon)

Both questions help the patient and family frame change as a positive movement, rather than a negative movement – giving up a habit. People more easily move toward a positive goal. If a patient frames the change negatively she can be asked:

"What will you do instead of (overeat, smoke)?"

"How would that benefit your life?"

Miller and Rollnick have accumulated an abundance of evidence that motivational interviewing impacts not only patients with addictions but also those needing to make other lifestyle changes. Researchers are gathering evidence in medical settings. Significant challenges remain. Physicians spend less time than counselors during their visits discussing lifestyle changes and receive little training in counseling techniques. Yet, preliminary studies reveal positive outcomes with motivational interviewing in medical settings as well [17].

One structure for incorporating motivational interviewing principles into pediatric well-child care involves the use of the four Cs, a mnemonic for: *Contact, Contract, Check-out, Commitment*. Let us look at how the four Cs might be used to provide anticipatory guidance with SIDS prevention. The national rate for noncompliance with the AAP recommendations is ~24% (1996) and much higher among poor families [18].

First, make emotional ***contact*** with the family (See Chap. 2).

The second step involves the physician asking the family for an agreement or ***contract*** to discuss safety and SIDS prevention. In a typical well visit, contracting means setting an agenda. During the first well-child the resident might say:

> "The AAP recommends pediatricians talk to all families about infant safety, including the prevention of Sudden Infant Death Syndrome, what we abbreviate as SIDS. Would you be willing to discuss this?"

If a parent says no, the process is stopped at that point. There is no coercion. If a parent says yes, then it is expected that both the physician and the parent will contribute to the discussion as partners.

> "Tell me what you know about preventing SIDS. What are you doing in this regard?" *Contracting allows for collaboration and avoids the resistance that stems from a parent being told what to do.*

Checking out, the third C in the mnemonic, refers to the process of uncovering any misperceptions a parent might have adopted. The clinician highlights discrepancies between a parent's goal to keep his or her baby safe with actual practices that might endanger the baby. Common *misperceptions* include:

- Infants will choke or strangulate in the supine position (Some parents place their babies prone or on their side as a result.)
- Infants can be monitored safely when close to the parent in the parent's bed.
- The best way to calm a crying infant is to keep the baby in the bed next to a parent.

A parent's misperceptions must be resolved before she will take in accurate information from the physician. The third person technique can help bring out a misperception when a parent does not do so spontaneously [19].

> "Lots of parents worry about their baby strangulating or choking when the baby is on his back. Is that true for you?"

> "Lots of parents hear about SIDS and want to make sure they keep their baby safe. They bring the baby into their bed to keep an eye on him. Is that true for you?"

> "Lots of parents want to make extra sure their baby feels comforted. When the baby cries they bring him into bed next to them. Is that true for you?"

The clinician helps the parent express the maladaptive belief or attitude so that it can be dealt with directly. The clinician then offers corrective information.

> "It's clear you are working real hard to make your baby safe. Would you be willing to hear information we have learned in extensive studies on sleep position?"

Once the parent agrees, the physician shares *accurate* information based on extensive research:

- Supine position on a firm mattress is the safest position for infants [20].
- Infants are at no more risk to *choke* in the supine position than the prone position [21].
- Approximately one-half of SIDS deaths now occur in parental beds [22].
- Attachment refers to a sturdy biological process that is not undone by brief periods of infant crying [23].
- A number of ways exist for parents to nurture and comfort babies without bringing them into bed. Once the physician shares the information, a parent confronts any discrepancy between her goal (e.g., keeping baby safe) and actual behaviors (baby in parent's bed).

The final C stands for a ***commitment*** to a plan of action. The parents are asked if they are ***willing*** to follow the AAP guidelines on SIDS prevention. They are not asked ***to try***. (Some plans of action for families will be more extensive than simply following the AAP guidelines. Some may involve referral to other organizations: parenting groups; Weight Watchers; individual counseling, etc. Others may involve frequent pediatric visits.) In the previous example, Gottman affected change in couple relationships only after he implemented a six-step plan in a structured series of meetings run by him and his wife, as co-therapist [12]:

Clinician: If I am hearing you right, you want to use the back position to put Emily to sleep because you believe the safety recommendations. Only, you believe that Emily is more comfortable on her stomach and sleeps better.

Mother: Yes, that's right.

Clinician: Would you be willing to experiment with putting Emily down on her back for a minimum of one week if I teach you other ways of calming her, before you put her down.

Mother: Yes, I would be willing. (Table 6.1) (Harvey Karp, M.D. describes very effective comforting techniques in *The Happiest Baby on the Block*.)

TABLE 6.1. Four Cs

Contact	Emotional contact leads to relationship building. All the skills we discussed in Chap. 2 apply: friendliness, tracking, empathy, and positive regard.
Contract	Agreement between family and physician regarding their work together. The contribution of each is made clear in order to promote a successful outcome.
Checkout	Process of asking about family's understanding of the situation to uncover any misperceptions and provide accurate information.
Commitment	Will the family commit to a plan of action?

WELL-CHILD CARE

I propose the following structure for Jack, that second year resident doing well-child care. Before focusing on the four Cs, Jack must ask himself three basic questions. These three **developmental** questions regarding the child and family will help Jack frame the encounter.

1. What is the main psychosocial task of a child this age? What are the behaviors expected of a child accomplishing this task? [24]
2. How is this child doing with regard to the expected behaviors of a child in this development stage?
3. How is the family supporting this child in the progress?

The four Cs then provide the structure for offering the anticipatory guidance and behavioral counseling.

- Establish and maintain emotional *contact* with each member of the family.
- Agree to an overall *contract* for health supervision, as well as a specific contract for each session. If a family brings up a concern, the specific contract involves that concern. If a family expresses no particular goal for that session, a topic or topics can be introduced. The clinician prioritizes topics to suggest to the family for discussion based on the child's developmental stage and importance of the topic to the child's overall health (SIDS prevention is an important topic in the newborn period because SIDS is the leading cause of death in infants after 1 month of age.)
- *Check out* the family's thoughts and feelings about the issue. Identify family goals and values. Uncover any misperceptions and provide accurate information. Rate family's sense of confidence and conviction regarding change, if appropriate.

- Ask the family what they would like to do in view of the new information. Ask for a *commitment* to a plan of action (e.g., a change in family behavior; a return appointment for further assessment). Of course, the family may opt to commit only to think about the matter, perhaps to discuss it further with you at a future visit.

The clinician organizes the well-child visit, moving flexibly between the steps. The clinician establishes emotional contact at the same time he assesses the child and family's functioning. We will look at a case example to make this structure come alive.

SIX MONTHS WELL-CHILD VISIT USING 4C METHOD

Mia, a 6-month-old baby in for her checkup, looks like a Gerber baby. Her parents appear delighted with her. They express no concerns. The pediatrician structures the visit using the above approach. He asks himself three questions at the beginning of the visit.

- What is the main developmental task (with associated behaviors) of a 6-month-old?
- How is Mia doing with these tasks?
- How is the family supporting Mia in achieving the task?

A 6-month-old baby is transitioning to a new stage (see Table 6.2). Having developed a secure base as a result of consistent and loving care giving, a 6-month-old baby will soon be exploring everything in her environment. The baby is in love with the world. Mia, supported by her parents as she transitions into the exploring stage, is progressing beautifully. The pediatrician affirms the parents and increases contact with them.

TABLE 6.2. Structure for well-child care

Clinician asks self
  What is the main psychological task of a child this age?
  How is this child progressing with regard to the expected behaviors of a child in this developmental stage?
  How is the family supporting this child's movement through this stage?
As clinician
  Establishes and maintains emotional *contact*/build a relationship
  Agrees to a *contract* for the session and their work together
  Checks out family's thoughts and feelings:
    Clarifies and makes explicit family's ambivalence
    Clears up misperceptions
  Asks for a *commitment* to a plan of action, if appropriate

Pediatrician:	You really enjoy Mia. She is responding wonderfully to your nurturing. She looks secure and ready to explore her environment. Do you have questions about how to support Mia during this stage.
Parent:	We have baby-proofed the house so she can scoot around, play with the pots and pans. The pediatrician reviews the specifics of baby-proofing the house, affirming the parents once again in the process. He then asks them for a contract.
Pediatrician:	Do you have any questions about Mia or her next stage of development?
Parent:	No. She seems to be doing well.
Pediatrician:	Would you like to spend a few minutes talking about sleep habits? A lot of recent research highlights the importance of good sleep habits. In my experience babies often change their sleep habits in this next stage.
Parent:	That sounds fine.
Comment:	The pediatrician could have asked about any number of topics recommended by the AAP. He has been intrigued by recent articles describing negative consequences of sleep deprivation on attention and emotional regulation. He knows that as infants begin to differentiate in the next 6 months, they often have sleep disruptions, a manifestation of separation anxiety. He asks their understanding and feelings.
Pediatrician:	Tell me what your bedtime routine is like?
Parent:	We give Mia a bottle and then I rock her to sleep. It takes about 20–30 minutes, although sometimes she won't go to sleep.
Pediatrician:	Does she sleep through the night?
Parent:	Usually she wakes up a couple of times. I go back and rock her to sleep.
Pediatrician:	You comfort her nicely.
Parent:	Thanks.
Pediatrician:	I can think of only one problem with that approach. Mia associates being rocked and falling asleep.

So when she wakes up, as all babies do, she tries to recreate the initial association and cries until you rock her back to sleep. Would you be interested learning how you can change that?

Parent: I don't want to let her cry and feel I've abandoned her.

Pediatrician: Of course not. So you worry that if you allow her to cry and calm herself, the secure base you have established with her will be damaged.

Parent: Yes, I don't want to risk that.

Pediatrician: Well, you really won't be risking that. We know that a strong biological force like attachment is not damaged by occasional periods of a baby crying. The overall pattern of providing warmth and being attuned to a baby determines how a baby attaches.

Parent: I believe that. It just would be hard to hear her cry.

Pediatrician: I imagine it would be hard. I can teach you a progressive method that is fair to your baby. Are you interested in that?

Comment: The pediatrician again asks for a new contract. If the family says yes, he can provide them appropriate information. We notice the pediatrician smoothly move through the steps. Several times he moved back to check their understanding or their thoughts and feelings on the subject. In the end, the family may or may not want to commit to a plan of action.

CAPACITY

The problem of the clinician's time limits and his capacity to include all the recommended topics remains unresolved. A number of excellent topics for anticipatory guidance have been ignored (see Appendix D for a brief discussion of capacity).

Before we finish our discussion of well-child care, let us return to Jack. Jack was that discouraged second year resident in continuity clinic facing a tough psychosocial problem. Using the above well-child structure, Jack reviews Braxton's progress with regard to the main task of a 7-year-old; develop competence socially with peers and academically in school. He recognizes that Braxton has difficulty with all lines of development – physical, cognitive, emotional, and social. He will continue to use the 4C structure.

TABLE 6.3. Developmental tasks

0–6 months	Develop basic trust and a solid attachment through mirroring admiration[a]
6–12 months	Explore and experiment (Love affair with the world)[a]
1–3 years	Achieve a sense of *Okayness* as an autonomous individual, having his own wants, feelings, and thoughts. Separate feelings from thoughts and actions and begin to learn to control his impulses. *You can be as angry as you want. The bottom line is you can't hit your sister.*
3–6 years	Use imagination to master his world. Develop sense of self as an individual *I'm a boy; I'm good at kicking the soccer ball; my friend is Timmy.* Manage transition to school
7–10 years	Negotiate demands/routines outside the family. Develop competency in academics, with friends, and in activities
11–13 years	Identify with peer group while taking independence from family
14–16 years	Learn responsibility for managing own needs, feelings, and behaviors. Achieve sexual sense of self and separate sex from nurture
17+ years	Achieve mature sense of self – relationships, values, vocation

Successful completion of early tasks forms foundation of later tasks.
[a]Description from Louise Kaplan [25].

Only, his purpose now will be to ask for a commitment to mental health referral, since the complexity of Braxton's problems is beyond the scope of a general pediatric practice.

Recommended Reading: *Encounters with Children*, 4th ed. by S. Dixon and M. Stein (Table 6.3).

References
1. Wood D (2003) Effect of child and family poverty on child health in the United States. Pediatrics 112:707–711
2. Regaldo M, Halfon N (2001) Primary care services promoting optimal child development from birth to three years: review of the literature. Pediatr Adolesc Med 155:1311–1327
3. Moyer VA, Butler M (2004) Gaps in the evidence for well-child care: a challenge to our profession. Pediatrics 114:1511–1521
4. Yarnell KSH, Pollak KI, Ostbye T, Krause KM, Michener L (2003) Primary care: is there enough time for prevention, research and practice? Am J Public Health 93:635–641
5. Glascoe FP (2000) Early detection of developmental and behavioral problems. Pediatr Rev 21:272–279
6. Reynolds AJ, Temple JA, Robertson DL, Mann EA (2001) Long-term effects of an early childhood intervention on education achievement and juvenile arrest. JAMA 285:2339–2346

7. American Academy of Pediatrics (2001) Developmental surveillance and screening of infants and young children. Pediatrics 108:192–196

8. Kuo AA, Inkelas M, Lotstein DS, Samsan KM, Scher EL, Halfon N (2006) Rethinking well-child care in the United States: an international comparison. Pediatrics 118:1692–1702

9. Telzrow RW (1978) Anticipatory guidance in pediatric practice. J Contin Educ Pediatr 20:14–27

10. Green M, Palfrey JS (eds) (2000) Bright futures: guidelines for health supervision of infants, children and adolescents, 2nd edn. National Center for Education in Maternal and Child Health, Arlington, VA

11. Stott NCH, Rollnick S, Rees MR, Pill RM (1995) Innovation in clinical method: diabetics care and negotiating skills. Fam Pract 12:413–418

12. Gottman JM, Gottman JS (2007) And baby makes three: the six-step plan for preserving marital intimacy and rekindling romance after baby arrives. Three Rivers Press, New York, NY

13. Rollnick S, Heather N, Bell A (1992) Negotiating behavior change in medical settings: the development of brief motivational interviewing. J Ment Health 1:25–37

14. Miller WR, Rollnick S (2002) Motivational interviewing: preparing people for change, 2nd edn. Guilford Press, New York

15. Keller VF (1997) Kemp-White. Choices and changes: a new model for influencing patient health behavior. J Clin Outcomes Manag 4:33–36

16. Platt FW, Gordon GH (2004) Field guide to the difficult patient interview, 2nd edn. Lippincott Williams &Wilkins, Baltimore, MD

17. Van Wormer JJ, Boncher JL (2004) Motivational interviewing and diet modification: a review of the evidence. Diabetes Educ 30:404–416

18. Brenner RA, Simons-Morton BG, Bhasker B, et al (1998) Prevalence and predictors of the prone sleep position among inner-city infants. JAMA 280:341–346

19. Gould RK, Rothenberg MD (1973) The chronically ill child facing death – how can one pediatrician help. Clin Pediatr 12:447–449

20. American Academy of Pediatrics Guidelines and Policies (2006) A compendium of evidence-based research for pediatric practice, 6th edn. AAP, Elk Grove Village, IL

21. Hunt L, Fleming P, Golding J (1997) ALSPAC Study team: does the supine sleeping position have any adverse effects on the child? I. Health in the first six months. Pediatrics 100:1–14

22. Blair PS, Sidehothan, Berry PJ, Evans M, Flemining PJ (2006) Major epidemiological changes in sudden infant death syndrome: a 20 year population based study in the UK. Lancet 367:314–319

23. Rutter M (1979) Separation experiences: a new look at an old topic. J Pediatr 95:147–154

24. Rothenberg MD (1974) The unholy trinity: activity, authority and magic. Clin Pediatr 13:870–873

25. Kaplan L (1978) Oneness and separateness: from infant to individual. Simon and Schuster, New York

7

Primary Care and Child Mental Health

*Mental illness, including suicide, accounts for over 15 percent of the burden of disease in established market economies, such as in the United States. This is more than the disease burden caused by **all** cancers.*

NIMH Statistics

Mary, a timid, sweet 8-year-old girl, has vomited intermittently over the last 2 weeks, but only on school mornings. She will not eat on school mornings, cries, says her belly hurts and that she cannot go to school. She has missed 4 days of school. Mary experienced difficulty separating in kindergarten and first grade, but those exacerbations were milder and quickly resolved. She will not visit her friends at their houses. Mary often comes into her parents' bed during the night. Her mother worries about her poor appetite and abdominal pain. The pediatrician has known the mother, Mrs. Heinz, for years and notes that Mrs. Heinz frequently worries about her children. Now, Mary worries. Mary worries that her mother may die while she is at school. Her mother tries to reassure her, but Mary is not reassured. Her father thinks she just needs to "get over it." Mary has Separation Anxiety Disorder and Functional Abdominal Pain [80% of children with Functional Abdominal Pain exhibit anxiety [1].]

Fifteen percent of children seen in a general pediatric practice experience clinical anxiety [2]. Children with anxiety are only a third as likely to be treated as are children with ADHD [3]. Anxiety and depression in children, called the internalizing conditions, are commonly *hidden* diagnoses since children may be unaware

J. Binder, *Pediatric Interviewing: A Practical, Relationship-Based Approach,* Current Clinical Practice, DOI 10.1007/978-1-60761-256-8_7, © Springer Science+Business Media, LLC 2010

of the meaning of their symptoms or may not want to talk about their symptoms because they might appear weak and vulnerable [4]. History must, therefore, be gathered from multiple (child, parent, teacher) sources [5]. Anxiety and depression contribute to unhealthy lifestyles, <u>such as</u> overeating and smoking, interfere with the management of chronic conditions such as asthma, frequently persist into adulthood, and lead to negative emotional and social sequela [6, 7]. The USA has experienced an increase in the frequency and severity of mental health conditions in children in the last two decades [8], at a time when child mental health resources in many parts of the country remain sparse (e.g. rural) [4]. Understandably, the American Academy of Pediatrics places a priority on pediatricians' recognition of emotional and social problems in children [9]. Pediatricians, however, seldom feel adequately prepared to take on this task [10].

The AAP expects pediatricians to recognize mental health conditions in children and to feel comfortable doing adequate mental health assessments (see Tables 7.1 and 7.2). Misdiagnosis and maltreatment result from improperly done evaluations (e.g. a preschool child who is hyperactive, secondary to family violence, can be easily misdiagnosed as <u>having</u> ADHD if the assessment is not thorough). *An adequate mental health assessment includes the HPI, medical history (symptoms of primarily biological illnesses, such as insomnia and fatigue, can overlap with mental conditions [11]), developmental, family, and social history. In addition, the pediatrician must have an understanding*

TABLE 7.1. Clues to the diagnosis of anxiety disorders in children and adolescents

Behavioral clues
  Hyperactive behavior
  Irritability/tantrums/defiance
  Freezing up
  Avoidance of social situations, school
Physical symptoms
  Headache/abdominal pain/sleep problems
Thinking characteristics
  "I can't do it"/"I can't handle" – sense of incompetence when child is capable of task
  "It's too hard"
  Difficulty concentrating
  Perfectionism/inflexibility
  Frequent *what if* questions/catastrophic thinking

TABLE 7.2. Characteristics – depressed children

Preschool
— Have "no fun"/bubble is burst [20]
– Restless/sleep problems [20]
– Thinking content – themes of death may be present [20]
Children and adolescents
– Weepy (sad), irritable, or bored mood [11]
– Difficulty with relationships [11]
– Hypersensitivity to perceived criticism [21]
– Separation anxiety/phobias [21]
– Somatic complaints (abdominal pain; headaches…) [22]
– Withdraw from favorite friends or activities [22]
– Slowed thinking or concentration [22]
– Negative view of self and others
– "I do everything wrong" – "Nobody loves me" –"I hate myself" [14]
– Neurovegetative symptoms and signs (appetite and sleep changes; e.g. staying up very late…) [22]
– Behavioral symptoms – aggression, truancy [22]

Depressed children are often *reactive* to changes in their environment and do not demonstrate the persistent melancholy of some depressed adults [22].

of mental health conditions and make inquiries of disorders that can mimic or co-exist with the primary diagnosis, and performing a mental status exam. Although pediatricians face a formidable task, it is the current standard of care. In the last decade, the numbers of children and adults with mental health conditions receiving treatment from primary care providers tripled [12].

Anxiety and depression have clearly been shown to be treatable conditions [13, 14]. Pediatricians must decide whether they will screen everyone for psychosocial problems or utilize surveillance (see Chap. 6). Although screening identifies children with psychosocial ailments much better than surveillance, some pediatricians do not consider screening feasible for their practices. Pediatricians who use surveillance inquire about anxiety and depression when children present psychosocial impairments or live in high-risk families. We now turn our focus to specific interviewing strategies that can help the primary care clinician uncover anxiety and depression in children. A thorough discussion of anxiety and depression in children, beyond the scope of this book, can be found in *Child and Adolescent Psychiatry: A Comprehensive Textbook* [14].

We will end the chapter by discussing how a clinician can make an effective referral to a mental health specialist. *What interview strategies help the pediatrician uncover childhood anxiety and depression?*

INTERVIEWING STRATEGIES FOR PRIMARY CARE PHYSICIANS

1. The physician considers the possibility of a mental condition even when the family does not voice a concern. The clinician has two areas to search for clues:

   - Behavioral red flags (e.g. frequent need for reassurance, unable to enjoy activities, avoidance of activities) [7]
   - Family patterns characteristic of anxious and depressed families (e.g. perfectionist, critical, rejecting, over protective) [15]

2. The clinician establishes a safe atmosphere for the child and family to talk – given a common reluctance to talk about mental health problems, including anxiety and depression in the first place.

   - She maintains a sound engagement through the use of non-verbal and verbal empathy, non-judgmental attitude, and a positive regard for the child and family.
   - Allows enough time for the discussion so that the family believes the clinician wants to hear the story.
   - Goes at a slow pace with anxious and depressed children. They frequently judge themselves negatively for having anxiety or depression. Going slow provides time for the child and family to trust that the clinician is on their side.
   - Begins the conversation on a topic the child is willing to discuss, such as a favorite hobby or daily activities.
   - Agrees to a clear agenda for the session. This leads to effective problem-solving and avoids pitfalls. "Recurrent abdominal pain in children can be due to stomach problems, urinary causes, emotional stress. Today, I will be asking about all those areas. Is that Okay?"

3. The clinician adopts a family perspective. As we discussed in Chap. 5, children form part of an interactive, dynamic system – the family. Parents both impact a child's manifestation of anxiety and depression and are impacted by a child's anxiety and depression. For instance, a parent might begin to hover and act irritated in response to a child's depressive withdrawal. The parents' hovering and irritability in turn worsen the child's depressive thinking. The circular process is completed with the parent feeling increased worry. The negative cycle becomes part of the data base needed for an adequate assessment and ultimately for treatment.

   Physician: When Mary goes to her room and shuts out everyone, what is that like for you?

   Mother: I feel awful.

Physician: Tell me what you mean

Mother: I feel so sad. I just want to give up.

Physician: Say more.

Mother: I don't know what to do to help her.

Physician: Mary, tell me what it is like when you see your mother get quiet.

Mary: I feel like I must be doing something wrong.

Physician: Tell me more about that.

Mary: I just feel bad…

Physician: It sounds like you and mom are in the same place. You know, feeling bad and withdrawing.

4. The clinician employs a variety of questioning approaches to enhance data collection since these children and families may exhibit a reluctance to talk. At least six types of questions can help carve out the topics of anxiety and depression (see Chap. 5 – *social history*).

Questions regarding the *impact* of anxiety and depression on daily functioning at school, at home, and with friends are essential.

"Mrs. Thompson, does Mary's worrying affect her academic performance?"

"How about friendships?"

This information allows the practitioner to determine whether the child's symptoms are related to a developmental stage or are symptomatic of a clinical condition.

Normalization, specifically the third person technique, helps uncover anxious or depressed feelings and behaviors [16].

"Lots of kids wonder if the other kids like them. Is it true for you?"

"Lots of children feel nervous when their mother goes to work. Is that true for you?"

Circular questioning can be used to assess family relationship patterns that might be maintaining and reinforcing the child's anxiety or depression [17].

"So, Mrs. Heinz, when Mary is crying and fearful about going to school, what happens inside you? What do you think? What do you do?"

"Mary, what do you think when mom tells you that you will be okay at school? What do you do?"

Many anxious children and families are compliant and respond to a *gentle command* with a deeper elaboration of the subject matter.

"Mary, tell me what you think when dad is late."

"Describe homework time in your house."

Empowering questions help a patient/family experience how the child is getting herself worried by her self-talk.

"Mary, how do you scare yourself about tests?"

"Mary, what do you say to yourself to get yourself upset about friends?"

It is important for Mary and her family to understand how Mary is creating her own worry [18]. If Mary is creating her own worry, then she can learn to stop worrying herself. This type of question would not be appropriate if she was not creating her own worry, such as with trauma. The use of language can help a child and family experience their personal power and own responsibility for changing their lives [19]. This concept can intrigue families and help promote active participation in the interview process when it is conveyed empathically.

Focused or detailed questions are needed to support a diagnosis and differentiate it from other conditions. Often, more than one condition is diagnosed. Formulating a differential diagnosis for mental health disorders needs to be as carefully done as is done for physical conditions. *The clinician asks for the descriptors of the symptom (e.g. anxiety) just as she does for physical symptoms like cough.* Questions that are helpful in differentiating conditions must be learned and asked (see Chap. 3). For example, a clinician differentiating ADHD from anxiety will be aware that ADHD typically presents signs by the preschool years while anxiety conditions manifest at different ages throughout childhood – *chronology descriptor* [7]. Valid screening instruments can help pediatricians develop familiarity with questions that help identify *specific* anxiety and depressive disorders. Even if the clinician does not use them as screens, she can learn what questions help uncover depression, separation anxiety disorder, social anxiety, etc. by keeping them available and referring to them periodically.

Center for Epidemiological Studies – Depression Scale – available at http://www.moodykids.org

Mood and Feelings Questionnaire – available at http://devepi. mcduke.edu/mfq.html

Screen for Child Anxiety-Related Emotional Disorders – SCARED: see Appendix E

Multidimensional Anxiety Scale for Children – MASC – author John March. The child versions of these screens have examples of simple and developmentally appropriate questions to ask.

We now return to Mary, the anxious 8-year-old girl, being evaluated by the pediatrician for recurrent abdominal pain. The pediatrician decides that she needs more information to make a better assessment. She schedules a family meeting to consider a mental health referral.

Excerpt (The pediatrician has already joined with all three family members.)

Dr. Murphy:	So it sounds like we all agree to spend this time talking about Mary's difficulty going to school
Mrs. Heinz:	And her anxiety in general.
Dr. Murphy:	Anything else?
Mrs. Heinz:	No, that's it.
Dr. Murphy:	Mr. Heinz, we have not heard your perspective yet. Would you tell us your thoughts and concerns?
Mr. Heinz:	I don't think Mary has any major underlying problem. She makes straight A's. She has friends. She is a great kid. I do feel very upset when she cries with her belly hurting and won't eat in the morning. We have tried reassuring her and that doesn't work. I think she just needs to go to school.
Dr. Murphy:	Mary what do you think?
Mary:	I want to go to school. My belly really does hurt.
Mrs. Heinz:	We believe you, honey.
Dr. Murphy:	Mr. and Mrs. Heinz, how do you decide how to handle this?
Mrs. Heinz:	That's the problem. We haven't decided. Sometimes we make her go to school and other times we give in.
Mr. Heinz:	Its not easy to decide what to do. When Mary is really crying hard we end up quarreling with each other.

Dr. Murphy:	That's an important point. If you haven't agreed how to handle the situation as a parenting team beforehand, the upsetment in the morning can lead to inconsistency, which increases Mary's anxiety. Would the two of you be willing to talk and decide how you want to handle this. Mary and I will just watch. Okay, Mary?
Mary:	Okay.
Mr. Heinz:	I think we need to be firm. Remember, she had the same problem last year and she got over it quickly.
Mrs. Heinz:	Well, I agree she needs to go to school consistently. I think we need to make sure she is not really sick first.
Mr. Heinz:	Dr. Murphy said she has functional pain. We know that.
Mrs. Heinz:	I know, but she could come down with something else too.
Mr. Heinz:	How about we ask Dr. Murphy to give us specific criteria to keep her home or bring her in to get checked.
Mrs. Heinz:	Okay.
Mr. Heinz:	One more thing. Earlier, you mentioned the possibility of going for counseling. I don't think she needs counseling. She is a normal child.
Mrs. Heinz:	I just don't want her to grow up anxious like me. Look how she becomes frightened if we mention getting a sitter.
Dr. Murphy:	Let me jump in and ask a few specific questions. I would like to ask questions about other anxiety and depressive conditions, just to be thorough. We will come back to the question of a counseling referral. Okay?
Mr. and Mrs.	Heinz: Okay
Comment:	Dr. Murphy decides to have Mary fill an anxiety questionnaire as she asks her parents questions about her mood.
Dr. Murphy:	Does Mary tend to get down on herself?
Mrs. Heinz:	Not at all.
Dr. Murphy:	Is she enjoying herself lately, playing with friends and doing activities?

Mrs. Heinz: Yes, nothing is changed in that area.

Comment: The following focused questions are examples of questions that can help Dr. Murphy identify and differentiate any other anxiety conditions. She already has identified Separation Anxiety Disorder. As her longtime pediatrician, she has accumulated medical, developmental, and family data. In addition, Mrs. Heinz requested a letter from Mary's teacher that she gives to Dr. Murphy. This data helps complete the data base.

Examples of focused questions

"Does Mary spend too much time doing things over and over or have to have things done an exact, certain way?" (looking for OCD)

"Do you consider Mary a worrier?"

"Does Mary worry about physical symptoms besides the belly pain?"

"Has Mary been exposed to any trauma?"

"How is Mary sleeping?"

"Is Mary able to concentrate well?"

Comment: After gathering the data, Dr. Murphy will decide whether to recommend a mental health referral.

MENTAL HEALTH REFERRAL

Families express more concerns about psychosocial issues than about any other category in a pediatric practice [23]. Since the research reveals that most mental health referrals fail, a thoughtful, careful process is indicated [24].The clinician must first decide which families to refer. A thorough understanding of the nature of the problem allows the clinician to make this decision. A clinician might treat a preschooler with misbehavior, but not if the primary issue was domestic violence.

In general, seasoned clinicians refer the following types of problems: ones that lie outside clinicians' expertise; the clinician's interventions have not worked; the family wants a referral; or the problems are too severe [25]. Severity is determined by assessing how many domains (school, family, and peers) are affected by the problem and the degree of functional impairment [25]. Sometimes families do not believe that a referral is necessary and the clinician wants to refer. In that instance, the clinician must go slow, respect the families' understanding and concerns, and work to help them see the problem from a new perspective [25]. We do better by empathizing with the patient's opinion ("Sounds like right now you both think a mental health referral would not be helpful. Did I hear that correctly?") and perhaps asking what might make them more amenable to that suggestion in the future so "we can be on the same page together."

The following *guidelines* support a smooth transition:

- The clinician gives herself enough time to fully discuss the referral [25].
- The problem, its impact on the child's functioning, and any interventions are reviewed.
- Since many families feel sensitive about a mental health referral, a normalization technique, such as the third person technique, can be helpful when the referral is made. "Many parents taking care of a challenging child with increased need for medical care, like Mary, have difficulty working as a team and find talking with a counselor with experience in that area helpful" [25].
- The clinician checks out how the family perceives the referral. "What do you think about what I just suggested—to go for counseling?"
- She explores any previous mental health experiences, and whether they helped.
- She helps the family understand the benefit of a referral in order for them to invest in it [25]. "Once the therapist helps Mary learn to talk out her feelings, she won't feel so desperate to get others to listen. She is likely to open up to you and lessen her disruptive behavior."
- The clinician provides specific information about the specialist, her approach, and insurance information [25]. When the primary care clinician and specialist collaborate, a smoother transition can be expected [25].

If the referral fails (family did not make or keep an appointment), the clinician explores this with the family [25].

"Would you be willing to talk about the referral for counseling we discussed last visit?"

A follow-up appointment helps the family understand that the primary care clinician is not "getting rid of them" [25].

I would like to schedule a follow up visit in three weeks. That will give you time to meet the specialist and decide if she is a good match for your family. When you return, I plan to recheck Mary's belly problem and her weight.

TABLE 7.3. Interviewing strategies for uncovering anxiety and depression in children in primary care

---

Observe for red flags
Create emotional safety – join with family – contract – start with nonsensitive
   topics/go slowly
Use of third person technique to move to emotional topics
Carve out anxiety/depression region with
   gentle commands
   circular questions – relationship patterns
   content-specific questioning to discriminate between conditions
     (Appendix C)
Impact of condition on academic and social functioning

MORE ABOUT MARY AND THE HEINZ FAMILY

The clinician obtained further information about Mary. She diagnosed Separation Anxiety Disorder and no other anxiety or depressive condition. Her separation anxiety caused mild social impairment (Table 7.3).

Dr. Murphy: Let me summarize. Mary has Separation Anxiety Disorder and no other anxiety or depressive conditions. Everybody agrees she is a thoughtful and delightful eight-year-old child who manages life well overall. She enjoys her friendships and does well in school. She has mild limitations because of her anxiety, not enough to suggest counseling. Mr. and Mrs. Heinz, you plan on working together to enforce school attendance consistently. Mrs. Heinz, you still carry some concerns about her developing chronic anxiety but want try to resolve your own anxiety and observe how things go for her.

References

1. Campo JV, Bridge J, Ehamann M et al (2004) Recurrent abdominal pain, anxiety and depression in primary care. Pediatrics 113:817–824
2. Benjamin RS, Costello EJ, Warren M (1990) Anxiety disorders in a pediatric sample. J Anxiety Disord 4:293–316
3. Chavira DA, Stein M, Barkley K, Stein MT (2004) Child anxiety in primary care: prevalent but untreated. Depress Anxiety 20:155–164
4. Tarshis TP, Jutle D, Huffman L (2006) Provider recognition of psychosocial problems in low-income latino children. J Health Care Poor Underserved 17:342–357

5. Birmaher B, Ryan N, Williamson DE, Brent DA, Kaufman J (1996) Childhood and adolescent depression: a review of the past 10 years. Part II. J Am Acad Child Adolesc Psychiatry 35:1575–1583
6. McDaniel SH, Campbell TL, Hepworth J, Lorenz A (2005) Family-oriented primary care, 2nd edn. Springer, New York
7. Chansky TE (2004) Freeing your child from anxiety: powerful practical solutions to overcome your child's fears, worries and phobias. Broadway, New York
8. Atladollis HO, Farner ET, Schendel D, Dalsguard S, Thomsen PH, Thomsen P (2007) Time trends in reported diagnoses of childhood neuropyschiatric disorders. Arch Pediatr Adolesc Med 161:193–198
9. American Academy of Pediatrics (2001) The new morbidity revisited: a renewed commitment to the psychosocial aspects of pediatric care. Pediatrics 108:1227–1230
10. Regaldo M, Holfen N (2001) Primary care services promoting optimal child development from birth to age three years. Arch Pediatr Adolesc Med 155:1311–1322
11. Brent DA, Birmaher B (2002) Adolescent depression. N Engl J Med 347:667–671
12. Wang PS, Lane M, Ofsen M et al (2006) The primary care of mental disorders in the United States. In: Manderscheid RW, Berry JT (eds) Mental health, United States, 2004. DHHS Pub. No. (SMA)-06-4195. Substance Abuse and Mental Health Services Administration, Rockville, MD
13. Freeman JB, Garcia AM, Leonard Hl (2002) Anxiety disorders. In: Lewis M (ed) Child and adolscent psychiatry: a comprehensive textbook, 3rd edn. Lippincott Williams and Wilkins, Philadelphia, PA
14. Weller EB, Weller RA, Rowan AB, Svadijan H (2002) Depressive disorders in children and adolescents. In: Lewis M (ed) Child and adolescent psychiatry: a comprehensive textbook, 3rd edn. Lippincott Williams and Wilkins, Philadelphia, PA
15. Garber J, Hilsman R (1992) Cognition, stress, and depression in children and adolescents. Child Adolesc Psychiatr Clin North Am 1:129–167
16. Gould RK, Rothenberg MB (1973) The chronically ill child facing death: how can the pediatrician help. Clin Pediatr 12:447–449
17. Kadis LB, McClendon R (1998) Marital and family therapy. American Psychiatric Press, Washington, DC
18. Janoff DS (1997) The treatment of panic disorder and agoraphobia. In: Lennox C (ed) Redecision therapy: a brief action-oriented approach. Jason Aronson, Northvale, NJ
19. McNeal J (1976) The parent interview. Trans Anal J 6:61–88
20. Luby JL, Hefflenfinger AK, Mrakotsky C et al (2003) The clinical picture of depression in preschool children. J Am Acad Child Adolesc Psychiatry 42:340–348
21. Birmaher B, Ryan ND, Williamson DE et al (1996) Childhood and adolescent depression: a review of the past 10 years. Part I. J Am Acad Child Adolesc Psychiatry 35:1427–1438
22. Shain BN, the Committee on Adolescence of the American Academy of Pediatrics (2007) Suicide and suicide attempts in adolescents. Pediatrics 120:669–676

23. Kelleher KS, McInerny T, Gardner ND, Childs GE, Wasserman RC (2000) Increasing identification of psychosocial problems. Pediatrics 105:1313–1321
24. Rushton J, Bruckman D, Kelleher K (2002) Primary care referral of children with psychosocial problems. Arch Pediatr Adolesc Med 156:592–598
25. Coleman WL (2001) Family-focused behavioral pediatrics. Lippincott Williams and Wilkins, Philadelphia, PA

8

Sensitive Topics: Suicidality, Child Abuse, Sexuality, Substance Abuse

In my experience, most errors in suicide assessment do not result from a poor clinical decision. They result from a good clinical decision being made from a poor or incomplete database.

Shawn Shea

Kenneth Cooper, MD, the father of aerobics, tells a story about a distraught, suicidal young man. This man decides to run until he falls dead of exhaustion. One day he goes for a long run. He does not stop until he collapses into a heap in New York City's Central Park. The only thing is that he doesn't die. He analyzes the situation and concludes that he just did not run hard enough. So, he tries again the next day. He runs harder. Again, he drops at the end of his running effort, but he does not die. Not discouraged, he tries again the third day. He experiences the same results. When he awakens the fourth day, he is amazed to discover he feels better. A runner is born.

This story of a runner highlights several important elements of adolescent suicidality. Adolescents often do not directly tell healthcare providers that they are having suicidal thoughts. Suicidal children and adolescents, just like this runner, can resolve their despair. The clinician must first identify their suicidal state in order to help them. If this runner had been taken to the emergency room when he collapsed with exhaustion, would the E.R. physician have uncovered the runner's suicidal intent? What approach would help this physician discover the runner's turmoil and suicidal planning?

J. Binder, *Pediatric Interviewing: A Practical, Relationship-Based Approach*, Current Clinical Practice, DOI 10.1007/978-1-60761-256-8_8, © Springer Science+Business Media, LLC 2010

In this chapter, we will put ourselves in the role of a physician evaluating an outpatient with hidden suicidal thinking. We will explore an approach that physicians can take to optimize the likelihood of uncovering these thoughts, based on Shawn Shea's *Suicide Assessment: A Guide for Mental Health Professionals and Substance Abuse Counselors*. Interviewing on sensitive topics like suicide necessitates skills that help the patient to share information with the interviewer, techniques often called "validity" techniques [1]. We will conclude the chapter with a brief discussion of other sensitive topics: child abuse, sexuality, and substance abuse.

SUICIDALITY

Suicide, the third leading cause of death in adolescents, is considered a *grave* concern by the American Academy of Child and Adolescent Psychiatrists [2]. The rate of suicide in adolescents has more than doubled over the last 50 years and has led to much more research in the last two decades [3]. The American Association of Suicidology, an organization dedicated to the understanding and prevention of suicide, notes the following:

- Over 90% of adolescents who commit suicide have suffered from a psychiatric disorder – depression, substance abuse, aggressive or disruptive behavior (conduct disorder) [3].
- Interpersonal difficulties precipitate most adolescent suicide attempts [4].
- 16.9% of students (based on the 2003 Youth Risk Behavior Surveillance Survey) seriously considered attempting suicide in the previous 12 months [5].
- Experts estimate that 100–200 attempts are made for every completed suicide by youth [6]. Clinicians experience difficulty predicting benign vs. ominous suicidal behavior. Mild attempters may eventually commit suicide [3].
- Each day there are approximately 11 youth suicides [4].
- Although deaths by suffocation (hanging) are increasing, firearms account for the majority of completed suicides [7].
- Gay, lesbian, and bisexual youth are more likely to experience suicidal thoughts and attempt suicide [3].

These facts may not help us know that an individual adolescent is suicidal. To make such clinical decisions, we need a *full and accurate database*. Shea states that most mistakes are made as a result of inadequate data collection or omissions, not bad decisions made from a complete database [1]. Several conclusions can be drawn from this point:

1. Establishing a strong engagement in order to obtain a full database takes on added importance when performing a suicide assessment. Since a hurried pace is likely to disengage the patient, it is important for a clinician to monitor his pace.
2. Important data include the patient's nonverbal signs (e.g., fidgetiness). Note taking interferes with being fully present to the patient.
3. Interviewing the patient a second time is warranted if the clinician believes his data are incomplete [1].

Establishing an atmosphere that supports emotional contact and safety to talk can be extraordinarily difficult with a patient who feels shame, harboring a suicidal secret. Many adolescents have strong negative convictions about their own suicidal thinking. Some believe suicidal thoughts represent a character weakness or signify that they are crazy; others see suicidality as a sinful or taboo subject; and many believe nobody can help them, so they see no purpose for sharing their secret [1]. Physicians also hold any number of beliefs and attitudes that may interfere with a good suicidal assessment.

Interfering Cognitions
Physicians, like adolescents, may consider suicide as a sign of weaknesses, craziness, or sin; they may consider suicide a taboo subject or the situation to be hopeless. A physician holding onto any of those beliefs will convey judgment or disapproval to the patient. Patients attuned to the nonverbal signals of clinicians, such as a disapproving face, fast pace, or change in the tone of voice, may experience disapproval and then remain alone with their secret, just like the runner at the opening of the chapter [1].

A second group of beliefs and attitudes, just as incapacitating as the first group, almost always remain covert. A physician who uncovers suicidal thinking or behavior will need to spend extra time and energy in order to properly evaluate and triage that child or adolescent [1]. In addition, appropriate mental health referrals can be difficult to access. A busy pediatrician might hope that his patient is not suicidal so he would not be required to spend the extra time evaluating the patient. Although a normal wish, it is damaging to convey this wish to an adolescent who is already ambivalent about sharing her secret. Shea lists other physician attitudes that interfere with a competent suicide assessment.

Clinicians want to avoid anxiety. No physician wants to worry about a patient when he finishes his workday and goes home to his family, worry that can be expected by a pediatrician who has triaged a suicidal adolescent in his office earlier that day [1]. Instead of fleeing from his anxiety, the clinician must use it to solve the problem. Two questions can help a clinician stay fully present to his patient during a suicidal assessment.

"What am I feeling right now?"

"Is there any part of me that doesn't want to hear the truth right now?" [1]

A physician establishes an atmosphere of safety by first doing a self-examination and resolving any internal biases. He must then help diminish the shame that many adolescents experience with suicidal thinking. This shame results from the deeply held convictions about suicidality. A direct confrontation of these beliefs usually leads to a defensive reaction and poor engagement. The clinician needs a softer approach. Shea suggests two specific strategies for addressing this shame and secrecy: setting the platform and use of validity techniques [1].

Setting the Platform

The more we understand our patient's suffering, the more engaged we can be with our patient. By talking about her suffering, the patient will be more likely to share her suicidal state as she tries to seek relief from a painful depression or a state of "crises, anger, anxiety, and hopelessness." [1] The interviewer enters into the patient's experience of pain and uses that as a gateway to ask about suicidality. Asking about suicidality in that context feels natural and not like the question has been "popped" [1]. This physician moves from exploring the topic of depression to suicidality:

Allison: My friends get on my nerves. Most of the time I just hang out in my room.

Clinician: What's that like?

Allison: I feel really bad. I'm all alone.

Clinician: Tell me about being alone

Allison: It feels like no one cares about me (looks sad). I don't have anyone to talk to besides my dog.

Clinician (*slows pace*): You feel alone. Tell me more about that.

Allison: I don't know. I cry sometimes. I feel so all alone. Even my best friend Shelly has abandoned me. She doesn't call me anymore.

Clinician: It sounds difficult. Lots of folks who feel alone and down in the dumps have thoughts of wishing their life was over. Is that true for you?

Allison:	Sometimes.
Clinician:	Have you thought of ending it all, of killing yourself?
Comment:	Ask directly about killing oneself or being suicidal – not just hurting oneself. This area is too important to have miscommunication about what the patient means.

Increasing Accuracy

In the next step, the clinician asks questions in a way that increases the likelihood of obtaining an accurate database. He avoids negative bias ("You're not suicidal, are you?") and uses *validity techniques*. Validity techniques both enhance accuracy and increase engagement when used gently [1]. Engagement grows stronger as shame diminishes. I think three validity techniques are particularly useful for a primary care physician interviewing a potentially suicidal adolescent: normalization, gentle assumption, and the behavioral incident.

Normalization

When children and parents learn that other people have a similar feeling or experience, demonstrated with the third person technique, their shame or embarrassment often lessens [8].

> "Lots of folks who feel depressed have thoughts of wishing their life was over."

Indeed, many average high school adolescents have considered suicide over the last year. Suicidal thinking grows with depression, increasingly so as the depression becomes prolonged and deeper [3]. In fact, one should be dubious about the credibility of a very depressed adolescent who denies any suicidal thoughts. We normalize by helping the adolescent understand that suicidal thinking is a common experience in the throes of a clinical depression. We can reasonably hope the adolescent will see that she is not *weak*, *crazy*, or a *weird* human being, but that she is very much like the rest of the human race and that the interviewer is willing to listen and talk about her experience.

The clinician above entered the affectively charged area of suicidality with Allison, the 15-year-old girl who seemed depressed, using depression as a gateway to ask about suicidal thinking.

> "Allison, many folks going through a down or depressed period have thoughts of ending their life. Has that been true for you?" (***Normalization***)

Gentle Assumption
Gentle assumption, a variant of normalization, means gently questioning as if the behavior or thought in question is occurring [9]. The clinician implies that the patient's behavior is expected. It decreases shame.

Clinician: Have you had thoughts of suicide?

Allison: Not really (implies she has had thoughts)

Clinician: What thoughts have you had? (**gentle assumption**)

Allison: "Well..."

Gentle assumption could act as a leading question for a patient trying to please the physician. Therefore, it should never be used when asking a child about trauma [1].

Behavioral Incident
Gerald Pascal, a psychiatrist, described the third validity technique. Pascal observed marked disparities between patient reports of their child experiences and the actual happenings. Patients often responded "fine" when asked to describe their childhoods, yet had suffered significant neglect and harshness. He coined the term behavioral incident to signify the act of uncovering facts of the story vs. patient opinion. The clinician obtains a chronological history of concrete, specific behaviors [10]. The interviewer asks for details of the story, including the patient's thinking, feeling, and behavior at the time. Probably the only drawback to using a behavioral incident involves the amount of time it takes.

   The Behavioral Incident is extremely useful in assessing suicidal thoughts or events. The clinician must know specifics: the frequency and extent of suicidal thoughts, whether the patient has acted on any thoughts (e.g., put a handful of pills in her hands or picked up a loaded gun), and what the patient thought would happen.

Case: David, an 11-year-old boy with conduct problems, has been saying nobody loves him. His mother reports that he ran into the street yesterday and almost got hit by a car. The clinician interviews David regarding his difficulty at home. He uses a behavioral incident to explore suicidality.

Clinician: David, tell me about what happened when your mother called you to come into the house yesterday:

David: I got mad.

Clinician: And, then what happened?

David: I said I wasn't going to come inside.

Clinician: What happened next?

David: Mom said "Yes you are."

Clinician: Then?

David: I said "No I'm not." I started to run.

Clinician: What were you thinking as you ran?

David: I'm going to get away from her.

Clinician: And then what did you do?

David: I ran across the street.

Clinician: What were you thinking was going to happen to you?

David: I thought I might get hit by a car.

Clinician: Did you want to get hit by a car?

David: No. I just wanted to get away.

The **behavioral incident** forms one component of a comprehensive strategy for eliciting suicidal behavior; called the CASE (Chrono-logical Assessment of Suicidal Events) approach, used by many mental health specialists [1] (see Appendix B). The interviewing framework that we have used to organize our inquiry into suicidal-ity can be applied to other sensitive topics – violence to others (child abuse, domestic violence), substance abuse, sexuality. That framework has three pillars: perform a self-examination for cogni-tions and feelings that might block inquiry into a sensitive area; set the platform; and judicious use of validity techniques.

We now turn our attention away from the assessment of violence directed inward to the assessment of a form of violence directed toward others – child abuse.

CHILD ABUSE

Shannon Clark, a third year pediatric resident, is called to the ER on a Saturday evening to evaluate a child who is suspected to be a victim of child abuse.

Case: Joshua, a 23-month-old toddler with a spiral fracture of his femur, lies on a stretcher in the Emergency Room. The nurse noticed a circular scar on his upper arm when she started an IV and questions the possibility of an old cigarette burn. The older of the two brothers, four-year-old Jeffrey, walks around the room. Olivia, Joshua and Jeffrey's mother, appears apprehensive. Her live-in boyfriend, Johnny, sits next to her.

Before entering the exam room, Dr. Clark checks in with herself. She asks herself what she is experiencing emotionally. She notices mild anxiety. In the past, she has felt anger and disgust with abusive parents. She is not aware of feeling angry or punitive. She will continue to monitor her feelings. Dr. Clark will attempt to be nonjudgmental and join with the family. She will try to view them as fallible human beings, not monsters. After introducing herself and meeting the family, Dr. Clark begins the interview. As she joins with them, she begins to set the platform for her inquiry into possible child abuse.

Dr. Clark:	I am Dr. Clark, a senior pediatric resident.
Olivia:	I'm Olivia Jarrell. This is Johnny.
Dr. Clark:	(shaking hands): Hi. What would you like to be called.
Olivia:	Olivia and Johnny.
Dr. Clark:	Dr. Jones asked me to see Joshua and evaluate his injury. I would like to hear your concerns and obtain background medical and family information so I can best make recommendations to Dr. Jones. Is that agreeable to you?
Olivia:	Sure.
Johnny:	I guess so. I just want Joshua to get good care.
Dr. Clark	Of course. Let's start with some background information.
Comment:	Dr. Clark obtains a general contract for the interview. This takes on particular importance when trust is an issue. Many families suspected of abuse have little trust in the medical or social system [11]. She then moves to a neutral area, background information. She begins the process of getting to know them and setting the stage. She does not just pop the question.
Dr. Clark:	Let's start with everybody's name, age and relationship to Joshua.
Olivia:	I'm Olivia. I'm 22 and their mom. Joshua is 23 months. Jeffrey is three years old. This is Johnny, my boyfriend. He is 21.
Dr. Clark:	Thanks. I' like to take a few minutes to get to know you. Tell me about yourself.
Olivia:	I spend my day with the children and the house.

Dr. Clark:	Tell me more about that.
Olivia:	I spend my day playing with them, feeding them, cleaning after them. I like doing it. They are my whole life.
Dr. Clark:	So, your children are your life. You spend all your time attending to them. Do you have any family living nearby who can help out and give you a break?
Olivia:	Not really.
Dr. Clark:	That sounds tiring.
Olivia:	I'm used to it.
Dr. Clark:	Okay. Johnny how about you? Tell me about yourself.
Johnny:	I work for a fast food restaurant.
Dr. Clark:	What's that like for you?
Johnny:	Okay. I'm an assistant manager.
Dr. Clark:	Assistant manager.
Johnny:	Yes, I have a lot of responsibility. I work a lot of overtime.
Dr. Clark:	Sounds like you are busy.
Johnny:	I am, between work, home and the two children.
Dr. Clark:	U-huh. How about Jeffrey and Joshua?
Olivia:	Jeffrey is my shy one. Joshua never met a stranger.
Dr. Clark:	Tell me what they like to do.
Olivia:	They like to jump off the couch and wrestle. They are typical boys.
Dr. Clark:	So, they are active little boys.
Johnny:	I'd say so.
Dr. Clark:	Let's shift gears now and talk about Joshua's overall health? Has he had any serious medical conditions?
Olivia:	No.
Dr. Clark:	Has he ever been hospitalized?
Olivia:	No.
Dr. Clark:	Does he take any medication?
Olivia:	He just finished amoxicillin for an ear infection.

Dr. Clark:	Let me go down a list of symptoms and check out his medical history more thoroughly.
Comment:	Clark does a review of symptoms including asking about previous trauma. She moves to the developmental history. Joshua is moving through the stage of separation/individuation. Dr. Clark, aware that discipline issues are frequent at this stage, will use this developmental theme and the distress parents can experience as a gateway (*platform*) for her inquiry into child abuse.
Dr. Clark:	You mentioned earlier that Joshua runs around and tends to get overexcited. Tell me more about that.
Olivia:	He is on the go all the time.
Dr. Clark:	On the go.
Olivia:	Yes. He wears us out.
Dr. Clark:	How do you mean?
Olivia:	I have to chase him so he doesn't get into things and hurt himself.
Johnny:	He's hyper.
Dr. Clark:	Johnny, some kids who are hyper like to be independent and do things themselves. They can be a little stubborn. Is that true for Joshua?
Johnny:	Joshua is stubborn.
Dr. Clark:	How do you handle his stubbornness?
Johnny:	We just explain the situation to him.
Dr. Clark:	And, if that doesn't work?
Johnny:	We might give him a spanking. We are not one of those types of parents who spoil their kids.
Dr. Clark:	Johnny, it can be tough when a toddler is stubborn. Have you had times when you felt you lost your patience? (**Normalization**)
Johnny:	Occasionally, just like any other parent would.
Dr. Clark:	Have you ever felt yourself cross the line and hurt him?
Johnny:	No. Never.
Dr. Clark:	How about you, Olivia. Ever lose your temper and do more than you intended?

Olivia: No. I just walk away if I get mad.

Dr. Clark: I appreciate you giving me all this background information. This might be a good point to switch our focus and find out more about Joshua's injury. Walk me through what happened. (**Behavioral Incident**).

Comment: Dr. Clark admits the child to the hospital and consults the child maltreatment team, telling Olivia and Johnny her concern that Joshua has been intentionally injured. Managing suspected child abuse, a highly sensitive and complex area, should involve individuals from social service and law enforcement. Experts recommend an interdisciplinary team approach. Team members who interview children need to be trained and experienced [12].

The Child Interviewer Must

1. Establish safety (e.g., possible abuser not present). The interviewer must stay aware of the child's vulnerability. The AAP has guidelines of how to do that for inquiries into both physical and sexual abuse [13].
2. Form a rapport with the child.
3. Take a developmental perspective, using age-appropriate language and cognitive skills.
4. Discuss confidentiality.
5. Conduct a nonbiased, noncoercive, and *nonrepetitive* interview.
6. Use open-ended questions followed by neutral probing questions when needed.
7. Help child express what took place in other ways, if they are reluctant to talk (e.g., drawing, etc.).
8. Use short, simple sentences and avoid the use of ambiguous pronouns.
9. Attend to the child's terminology.
10. Avoid leading questions [12].

Joshua, less than 2 years old, is too young to interview.

The parent interviewer must see the adults separately in order to obtain each partner's perspective. In addition, 50% of children who have been abused live with domestic violence as well [14]. The clinician cannot safely ask about domestic violence with the partner present. Once separated, a team member inquires about domestic violence. This same approach is used whether the parents are in the hospital or in a primary care setting.

Domestic Violence Inquiry

> "Violence has become so common between *couples* I see that I'm asking all adults in my practice the following question: 'In the past year have you been hurt, slapped, kicked or hurt in any other way by someone with whom you live or are close to?'" [15].

This three-step interviewing structure used for inquiries into sensitive topics such as suicide and violence toward others can be adapted for adolescent health promotion. Several commonly suggested anticipatory guidance topics for teens – sexuality and substance abuse – fall into the category of sensitive topics.

SENSITIVE TOPICS: ADOLESCENT SEXUALITY

Adolescents will discuss sensitive topics with their physician only when they trust the **confidentiality** of their revelations. Typically a primary care physician will talk with children without parents present for part of the visit starting around age 11. Confidentiality is discussed with the family then and repeated as appropriate.

> "Ben will take on more responsibility for his own health care as he gets older. I would like to talk with Ben alone for part of the visit, so that he has the opportunity to talk about anything that might be hard to talk about in front of parents. Of course, I would talk to your parents, Ben, if you tell me about something that is dangerous to your health or somebody else. Do you all agree to this?"

The American Academy of Pediatrics recommends yearly check-ups for adolescents with good risk assessment and anticipatory guidance as one important strategy for addressing the increasing psychosocial morbidity of adolescent health status in USA (suicide, substance abuse, sexually transmitted diseases, pregnancy) [16, 17]. Several excellent questionnaires (e.g., C-APS) are available to support pediatricians with this task [18].

Clinicians, who do not use questionnaires, can organize adolescent risk assessment with a popular mnemonic. HEADSS refers to home, education/employment, activities, drugs, sexuality, and suicide/depression [18]. The clinician starts with questions about home and school. Adolescents typically answer these questions freely, which allows for later movement to sensitive areas. One such area is sexuality. During the first of the three steps in a sensitive inquiry, the clinician performs a self-examination, scanning for any hidden cognitive blocks to a full, nonjudgmental assessment. For example, a young physician might think it is inappropriate to take a sexual history from an adolescent of the opposite sex who is not that much different in age. He might worry that he will appear intrusive and that the patient will react negatively. If the clinician does not stay aware, address, and resolve this issue, he might rush his pace or even appear mechanical to the patient. The patient, sensing his discomfort, will not produce a full and accurate history. That young clinician must stay aware that providing good comprehensive care includes a sexual history and that the physician–patient relationship forms a professional relationship, not a romantic one. He can maintain a clear boundary (e.g., having a nurse present). The clinician moves to the second step, setting the platform, after resolving any internal blocks, such as the one we just mentioned.

Setting the Platform
This clinician sets the platform by asking about friends.

Clinician:	Tell me about your friendships at school.
Mindy:	I've got several really good friends.
Clinician:	You've got several really good friends. (echoing)
Mindy:	Yeah. We all hang out at lunchtime. We eat at the same table.
Clinician:	Do you see your friends outside of school.
Mindy:	We're always together.
Clinician:	What do you like to do for fun?
Mindy:	Lots of times we just talk.
Clinician:	It sounds like your friendships are a high priority in your life.
Mindy:	That's true.
Clinician:	Lots of teenagers your age are beginning to have romantic relationships. Is that true for you?
Mindy:	Yes. I've been talking to someone.
Comment:	In the above example, the clinician introduced the topic of friends with a gentle command: "Tell me about your friends at school." Starting with a series of mostly closed-ended questions works more effec-

tively with a reluctant adolescent. This would allow her time to become comfortable with the interview [19]. For example:

Clinician: Tell me about your friends at school.

Mindy: They're okay.

Clinician: What do you and your friends like to do for fun?

Mindy: We usually are texting each other or are just hanging out.

Clinician: So you like to hang out and talk. What kind of activities do you like to do together?

Mindy: Sometimes we go to concerts

Clinician: What kind of music do you like?

Mindy: All types.

Clinician: Do you like oldies?

Mindy: They're okay.

Clinician: Those are my favorite. Let me see if I've heard correctly. You and your friends like to stay connected. You talk or text each other. Sometimes you go to concerts but mostly you just like to be together with your friends. True?

Mindy: Yes.

Clinician: Lots of teenagers your age are beginning to have romantic relationships. Is that true for you?

Normalization

The clinician then uses the third person technique during the conversation about friendships and romantic relationships to smoothly transition to the topic of sexuality. The discussion of friends and romantic relationships operates as a gateway to sexuality. It feels natural and normal to the patient.

> "Some folks in high school are starting to have an interest in boys or girls in a sexual way [17]. Is that true for you?"

Or

> "Some teenagers are beginning to have sex. Have any of your friends had any sexual experiences, including kissing, touching or sexual intercourse?" [20]

This last inquiry could be followed by:

> "How about you. Have you ever been sexually involved with anyone? [21]"

The clinician avoids confusion by avoiding asking if the adolescent is "sexually active." Many adolescents interpret "sexually active" in ways that would surprise and were not intended by the interviewer [20]. In addition, the above questions do not make assumptions about sexual orientation. A gay or lesbian adolescent is then more likely to open up to the clinician.

The clinician tracks with the patient's answers. If the teenage is having sex, the clinician can ask about the use of protection from pregnancy and sexually transmitted diseases. If the teenage is not having sex, he can be asked how he feels about that and affirmed for his decision. He can be offered the opportunity to discuss these topics whenever the teenager is ready to take in that information.

Another option for setting the platform is to ask about sexual development – menstruation; enlargement of testes. The clinician uses sexual development as a gateway to ask about sexual experiences, contraception, sexually transmitted diseases, sexual assaults, etc. [20]. The clinician might enter this sensitive area by commenting:

> "I ask all adolescents these questions in order to be able to provide good health care." (normalization.)

SUBSTANCE ABUSE SCREEN

The clinician's self-examination and setting the platform are performed in exactly the same manner for substance abuse screening. Again, the clinician uses normalization to increase validity:

> "Some teenagers experiment with alcohol, marijuana, or other drugs. Is that true for you and your friends."

Children with significant substance abuse problems are routinely missed in primary care if they are not screened. The adult CAGE questionnaire has low validity in adolescents [22]. The CRAFFT screen, developed at Boston's Children Hospital, has excellent validity and reliability as an adolescent screen [22] (Table 8.1).

We now have a plan and powerful tools to manage sensitive and difficult topics. In Chap. 9, we will expand our focus to another very challenging type of interview, giving bad news (Table 8.2).

TABLE 8.1. CRAFFT youth version

Have you ever ridden in a **C**ar driven by someone (including yourself) who was high or had been using alcohol or drugs?	Yes	No
Do you ever use alcohol or drugs to **R**elax, feel better about yourself, or fit in?	Yes	No
Do you ever use alcohol or drugs while you are by yourself **A**lone?	Yes	No
Do you ever **F**orget things you did while using alcohol or drugs?	Yes	No
Do your **F**amily or **F**riends ever tell you that you should cut down on your drinking or drug use?	Yes	No
Have you ever gotten into **T**rouble while you were using alcohol or drugs?	Yes	No

Scoring: 2 or more positive items indicate the need for further assessment.
© Children's Hospital Boston, 2001. All rights reserved.
Reproduced with permission from the Center for Adolescent Substance Abuse Research, CeASAR, Children's Hospital Boston.
For more information *contact info@CRAFFT.org* or visit *http://www.crafft.org*

TABLE 8.2. Three step method – sensitive topic inquiries

1. Interviewer performs a self-examination of thoughts/feelings that might block inquiry on a sensitive topic.
2. Set the platform. Be persistent in understanding patient's narrative.
3. Use techniques to enhance validity:
   (a) Normalization/third person technique
   (b) Behavioral incident
   (c) Gentle assumption

Based on *Suicide assessment for mental health professional and substance abuse counselors*.

References

1. Sheas SC (2002) The practical art of suicide assessment. A guide for mental health professional and substance abuse counselors. Wiley, Hoboken, NJ
2. American Academy of Child and Adolescent Psychiatry, American Academy of Psychiatry (2004) Joint statement from the American Academy of Child and Psychiatry and the American Psychiatric Association for the Senate Substance Abuse and Mental Health Services Subcommittee of the health, education, labor and pensions committee hearing on suicide prevention and youth: saving lives, March 3, 2004
3. American Academy of Child and Adolescent Psychiatry (2001) Practice parameters for the assessment and treatment of children and adolescents with suicide behavior. J Am Acad Child Adolesc Psychiatry 40(supplement):245–515

4. Berman AL, Jobes DA, Silverman MM (2006) Adolescent suicide: assessment and intervention, 2nd edn. American Psychological Association, Washington, DC
5. Eaton DL, Kann L, Kinchen SA, et al (2006) Youth risk behavior surveillance – United States, 2005. MMWR 55:1–108
6. Goldsmith SK, Pelmar TC, Kleinman AM, Bunney WE (eds) (2002) Reducing suicide: a national imperative. National Academy Press, Washington, DC
7. Centers for Disease Control and Prevention (2005) Web-based Injury Statistics Query and Reporting System (WISQARS) [online]. National Center for Injury Prevention and Control, Centers for Disease Control and Prevention (producer). http://wwwcdc.gov/ncipe/wisars
8. Gould RK, Rothenberg MB (1973) The chronically ill child facing death: how can the pediatrician help. Clin Pediatr 12:447–449
9. Shea SC (1998) Psychiatric interviewing: the art of understanding: a practical guide for psychiatrists, psychologists, nurses and other health professionals, 2nd edn. WB Saunders, Philadelphia, PA
10. Pascal G (1983) The practical art of diagnostic interviews. Dow Jones-Irwin, Homewood, IL
11. Newberger EH (1993) Child physical abuse. Primary Care 20:317–327
12. Sattler JM (1998) Clinical and forensic interviewing of children and families: guidelines for the mental health, education, pediatric and child maltreatment fields. Jerome M Sattler Publishers, San Diego, CA
13. American Academy of Pediatrics (2006) Guidelines and policies: a compendium of evidence-based research for pediatric practice, 6thn edn. American Academy of Pediatrics, Elk Grove, IL
14. Magen RH, Conroy K, Hess DM, Panciera A, Simon BL (2001) Identifying domestic violence in child abuse and neglect. Invest J Interpers Violence 16:580–601
15. Little KJ (2000) Screening for domestic violence: identifying, assisting, and empowering adult victims of abuse. Postgrad Med 108:135–141
16. American Academy of Pediatrics (2000) Committee on practice and ambulatory medicine. Recommendations for preventive pediatric health care. Pediatrics 105:645–646
17. American Academy of Pediatrics (2001) Committee on Psychosocial Aspects of Child and Family Health. The new morbidity revisited: a renewed commitment to the psychosocial aspects of pediatric care. Pediatrics 108:1227–1230
18. Maehr J, Felice M (2006). Eleven to fourteen years: early adolescence age of rapid changes. In: Dixon SD, Stein MT (eds) Encounters with children: pediatric behavior and development, 4th edn. Mosby Elsevier, Philadelphia, PA
19. McDaniel SH, Campbell TL, Hepworth J, Lorenz A (2005) Family-oriented primary care, 2nd edn. Springer, New York
20. Maehr J, Felice M (2006) Fifteen to seventeen years: mid adolescence – redefining self. In: Dixon SD, Stein MT (eds) Encounters with children: pediatric behavior and development, 4th edn. Mosby Elsevier, Philadelphia, PA

21. Friedman LS (2006) Seventeen to twenty-one years: transition to adulthood. In: Dixon SD, Stein MT (eds) Encounters with children. Pediatric behavior and development, 4th edn. Mosby Elsevier, Philadelphia, PA
22. Knight JR, Sherritt L, Shrier LA, Harris SK, Chang G (2002) Validity of the CRAFFT substance abuse screening test among adolescent clinic patients. Arch Pediatr Adolesc Med 156:607–614

9

Supporting Families Expressing Grief While Giving Bad News

*Listen to what they're saying. Care about it. Most times caring
about it is even more important than understanding it. Most
of us don't value ourselves or our love enough to know this. It
has taken me a long time to believe in the power of simply saying
"I'm so sorry," when someone is in pain. And meaning it.*

Rachel Naomi Remen

Case: David, a third year resident, enters the exam room for
Andrew's 2½-year-old well-child visit. His family recently joined
the clinic practice. Andrew is running around the room. He makes
fleeting contact with the adults in the room. He makes no spontaneous verbalizations. He seems to be driven by a motor. His
mother appears unaware of David's developmental problem or
the severity of the condition. David becomes aware that he does
not even want to be in the room with this family. He knows the
mechanics of how to give bad news. Only, he had not planned on
doing it this afternoon during his continuity clinic. Often the need
to give bad news cannot be anticipated. David does sit down to talk
to with Andrew's mother at the conclusion of the visit. The Ages
and Stages screening questionnaire identified Andrew as a child
who needs a comprehensive, developmental evaluation.

Resident: Mrs. Green, I would like to talk with you about the
               results of the developmental screen we gave Andrew
               today.

Mrs. Green: What did it show?

J. Binder, *Pediatric Interviewing: A Practical, Relationship-Based
Approach,* Current Clinical Practice, DOI 10.1007/978-1-60761-256-8_9,
© Springer Science+Business Media, LLC 2010

Resident:	We were hoping for a different result. It identified Andrew as falling outside the normal development of children his age.
Mrs. Green:	He'll be able to catch up, won't he?
Resident:	You are asking a very important question that I cannot answer today. I imagine it must be very difficult to not get a clear answer immediately.
Mrs. Green:	Well, I think he understands everything. He just doesn't talk yet.
Resident:	It sounds like you have noticed that Andrew is behind on his talking but he seems to understand well. What does your husband say about his talking.
Mrs. Green:	He has noticed that he doesn't talk much. He thinks his older sisters do too much for him, so he doesn't have to talk.
Resident:	So you have both noticed some difference from the way your daughters began talking. I would like to schedule a time this week to sit down with you and your husband to discuss what the screening results mean and look at the next step. Would that be okay with you?
Mrs. Green:	Sure.

The Accreditation Council for Graduate Medical Education lists the skill of giving bad news compassionately as an important part of a residency training curriculum [1]. Even third year medical students are expected to begin learning key elements of this complex skill [2]. Twenty years ago, giving bad news was not included in the curriculum of many medical school and residency training programs despite immediate and long-term negative consequences for the patient when bad news is delivered poorly [3].Why have we witnessed such a remarkable change? Two explanations make intuitive sense. The explosion of media coverage into every aspect of American life shifted the patient–physician relationship out into the public domain, to be analyzed and frequently criticized. The medical community responded to that criticism with a medical school curriculum change. In addition, a number of concrete recommendations for giving bad news have been endorsed by various authoritative organizations, based on the reports and studies of families given bad news [4]. These are readily teachable.

Learning how *to be* with a patient who is grieving or dying appears to be a bigger challenge than learning the mechanics of giving bad news, although both are important and intertwined. Physicians frequently find it difficult just *being* with grieving and dying patients, as opposed to *doing* for them [5]. It may be part of the legacy of modern, highly technical care. The portrait of the family doctor making a visit to the home of a dying patient and sitting with the family reflects an image from the distant past.

Clinicians consider staying present to grieving parents as particularly difficult. The potential loss of a child is the greatest loss a human can suffer. A parent who loses a child must grieve the loss of all her hopes and dreams for the future of that child, as well as for her own future that she had envisioned. In addition, she loses the opportunity to heal old wounds that she might have imagined would be resolved as a result of her child's life [6]. I will devote the first part of this chapter to the issue of staying emotionally present to these and other families facing bad news, before looking at expert recommendations for giving bad news.

STAYING EMOTIONALLY PRESENT TO FAMILIES

During the Marshall University Department of Pediatrics ongoing interviewing seminar for residents, we looked at the type of thoughts physicians express when faced with giving bad news. Resident endorsed the following concerns during one workshop of giving bad news:

"I might not say the right thing."

"I don't know how to explain everything."

"I might make a mistake and that would be terrible."

"I'm inadequate to the task."

"I wouldn't be able to handle it if the family has a huge reaction."

"I don't want them to blame me."

"I won't be able to handle it if they get angry with me."

"I can't deal with the potential loss of a child."

A physician holding any of these beliefs will be distracted. Many of these beliefs reflect *core* beliefs about self in relationship to others. Because negative core beliefs about self are often formed as a result of discouraging or hurtful childhood experiences, they are stored in parts of the brain that become activated by painful feelings such as anxiety or sadness [7]. Physicians commonly experience these painful feelings when faced with the task of giving bad news. Not uncommonly, clinicians attempt to avoid those painful feelings by busily trying to protect families from feeling badly. Sometimes, this attempt to avoid painful feelings is a reflection of unfinished grief from the clinician's own past, which has been triggered by the family's grief [6].

A brief exploration of several negative core cognitions will demonstrate that they are distorted or inaccurate, effectively blocking honest communication. A physician who must say it right or know everything is expressing a euphemism for "I must do it perfectly." In striving to reach that impossible and unreachable standard, the physician is not really able to listen to the patient. Instead, he is responding to an internal voice telling him to do it perfectly in order to be okay [8]. Yet, patients do not want perfect doctors. Survey after survey confirms that they want *good enough* doctors who are compassionate. Another statement from the seminar promotes a myth about feelings:

"They will have too big an emotional reaction."

The idea that feelings the patient expresses might be *too much* distorts reality. Babies are not born dampening down their feelings. They cry fully to communicate their needs. Only over time do they learn from the environment that certain feelings are too much [9]. Intense feelings are an appropriate expression of grief.

If the clinician examining his own thinking uncovers any thoughts or fears that are getting in the way of being present to the family, he addresses them. For example, if he realizes that he is trying to do it just right, he can remind himself that families want compassionate clinicians, not perfect ones.

The clinician then reviews recommended practical strategies for giving bad news.

RECOMMENDATIONS FOR GIVING BAD NEWS

The clinician should use a private setting, free of distractions. He arranges for coverage, so beepers or cell phones do not interrupt. All parties should be seated [4]. Both parents should be invited. Any relatives, like grandparents, who parents wish to be present, can be included [4]. Another health professional, such as a nurse, who knows the family well, might be helpful in the process. The clinician refers to the child by name. Barbara Korsch identified the importance of warmth and connecting with each member of the family. Patients express satisfaction when a physician connects with them person-to-person [10]. The clinician checks to see if the family is ready to talk. Experts frequently suggest helping a family prepare to hear bad news by firing off a *warning shot* [11].

> "The condition appears to be more serious than I first thought."

It is important for the clinician to be clear and straightforward. He should avoid vagueness and jargon. Families generally want to know the diagnosis as soon as the clinician makes the diagnosis [4]. As the clinician shares information, he is careful not to destroy hope for that family [4]. The way one family maintains hope is personal to that family and may be very different from another family. Time often helps a family change. Parents facing the loss of their child might pray for a miracle. Later, they might simply hope for a painless and peaceful death for their child.

The clinician takes a *slow pace* and pays attention to nonverbal signals from the family so that he does not overwhelm a family with information. For example, a family may focus on what seems to be an irrelevant detail as a way to signal that they are not ready to hear more at this point in time [4]. Some families need the information given in small chunks. That does not mean they need overly optimistic information. Inaccurate information prevents them from acknowledging and grieving their losses. I have witnessed parents of children holding onto a diagnosis of *developmental delay* describe their frantic efforts to help their child *catch up*, when the child appeared severely mentally retarded. An overly negative prognosis does not help families either. One study found that residents adopted a more pessimistic prognosis than faculty when talking with families in the Pediatric Intensive Care Unit [12]. No doubt some residents thought they were protecting the families from experiencing the disappointment of a bad outcome. Although these residents made their prognostic statements with good intentions, families cannot be protected from feeling the pain of loss.

One way for the clinician to monitor his pace is to check, and recheck, the family's understanding *throughout* the course of the meeting [4]. The clinician must avoid the temptation to focus solely on what can be done. Families want to know what it all **means** [13]. They may experience difficulty saying that clearly because of their own anxiety.

> "Let me check out what you have heard me say so far-to make sure I have said it clearly."

Of course, the clinician maintains an empathetic stance. The clinician observes nonverbal signals and elicits the family's *feelings*. The clinician tracks with the family's emotional response:

"You look sad"

"I can imagine that it must be heartbreaking to hear this news."

Some families protect themselves through a denial of the reality. It feels like it is too much to let in all at once. The clinician expresses empathy for these families by an acceptance of their denial. This state of shock is simply labeled.

"I imagine this information seems overwhelming – almost like a shock too hard to comprehend."

Other families express their sad, broken state, and stay open to receiving empathy (reflection, normalizing statements; hands held, etc.) from the clinician.

Vann Joines teaches a powerful intervention at the Southeast Institute for Individual, Group, and Family Therapy. He suggests a *feeling* response when a person is grieving and expressing feeling. Questions and statements that invite *thinking* responses often move clients away from heart-to-heart exchanges. Examples of thinking responses might be:

"Who will support you as you deal with this news?"

"It's natural to feel sad when you hear that your child has a chronic lung disease."

Talking about feelings can be educational and important. However, families move through the grief process by experiencing their feelings. Examples of feeling responses follow: (said softly)

"It's a big loss"

"It's painful"

"Breathe" (if they are holding their breath)

"Put words to your tears"

Silence for 5 to 30 seconds

I once saw a physician give a feeling response that captures the essence of this response. An elderly woman cried as Dr. Tim Campbell was making his morning rounds. The distraught woman described how she had not been allowed during the previous night to visit with her gravely ill husband of 50 years. Dr. Campbell responded with simple compassion. He hugged the woman. She calmed down and then they talked. I remember the incident because that woman was my mother.

TABLE 9.1. Giving bad news self-examination

Do a personal grief inventory, attending to one's own history of loss
  and grief
Self-talk that might interfere with being fully present to patient
Stay aware of own feelings in order to manage them and respond
  empathically to family
Expert recommendations
  Private setting/both parents
  Contract (agreement to meet)
  Give warning shot
  Empathy (*"I imagine..."*)
  Give news in chunks
  Check family's understanding and emotional response all along the way
  Go slowly
  Tell them what it *means*
  Arrange follow-up

Physicians can allow themselves to ***imagine*** what the family might be experiencing in order to respond with a feeling or heart-to-heart exchange. Although it can be painful to even imagine what a family is experiencing, a compassionate physician does just that. In a sense, the physician keeps one foot in the patient's experience and one foot out, because he cannot really feel the patient's pain. But, he can let them know he understands what they are experiencing by asking them what it is like for them to hear this news, responding with empathy, and staying silent as the family lets his statement register.

> "It looks like it is heartbreaking to hear this type of news about your child."

The flexible use of these guidelines allows for the unique needs of each family to be compassionately addressed. Studies show that families frequently do not remember much about the session other than the attitude of the physician [3]. Some clinicians record the session and give the tape to the family. Whether or not that is done, all families need a follow-up session. This allows the family to ask questions that have arisen and for the physician to check in on their emotional state. Any referrals or other specific information likely to be forgotten can be written down for the family (Table 9.1).

References

1. Accreditation Council for Graduate Medical Education (2005) Advancing education in interpersonal and communication skills: an educational resource from the ACGME outcome project. ACGME Outcome Project, Chicago, IL
2. Garg A, Buckman R, Kason Y (1997) Teaching medical students how to break bad news. CMAJ 156:1159–1164
3. Fallowfield L (1993) Giving sad and bad news. Lancet 341:476–478
4. Girgis A, Sanson-Fisher RB (1993) Breaking bad news: consensus guidelines for medical practitioners. J Clin Oncol 13:2449–2456
5. Remen RN (1996) Kitchen table wisdom. Riverhead, New York
6. Neimeyer R (2006) Lessons of loss: a guide to coping. Center for the Study of Loss and Transition, Memphis, TN
7. Beck JS (1995) Cognitive therapy: basics and beyond. Guilford Press, New York
8. Harris A (1972) Good guys and sweethearts. Trans Anal J III:1:13–19
9. Goulding MM (1997) Childhood scenes. In: Lennox CE (ed) Redecision therapy: a brief, action-oriented approach. Jason Aronson, Northvale, NJ
10. Korsch BM, Aley EF (1973) Pediatric interviewing techniques: current pediatric therapy. Sci Am 3:1–42
11. Buckman R (1992) How to break bad news: a guide for the health care professional. John Hopkins University Press, Baltimore, MD
12. Marcin JP, Pollack MM, Kuntilal MP, Sprague BS, Ruttinunn UC (1999) Prognostication and certainty in the pediatric intensive care unit. Pediatrics 104:868–873
13. Coulehan JL, Block MR (2006) The medical interview: mastering skills for clinical practice, 5th edn. FA Davis, Philadelphia, PA

10
Challenging Patients

Everyone in life has to climb unexpected mountains that were never wished for nor requested. A lucky few figure out how to enjoy the hike.

Foster Cline and Lisa Greene,

On a hot, muggy August day in Greece in the year 2004, a relatively unknown, but well trained, Brazilian runner, Vanderlei de Lima, led an elite pack of Olympic runners on the historic Marathon to Athens course. The messenger Phidippedes first ran that path over 2,000 years ago [1]. Six kilometers remained. People of all nationalities lined the streets screaming encouragement to Vanderlei. Suddenly, a deranged Irish cleric broke through the barricade, sprinted right to Vanderlei and literally tackled him to the ground. Vanderlei, naturally, experienced terror. With the help of a fan, Vanderlei broke loose, scrambled to his feet, and reentered the race. He lost his lead and a chance for the gold medal.

Vanderlei emerged from the stadium tunnel onto the track, now in third place. He joyfully celebrated his bronze medal by swinging his arms, imitating an airplane, and exhibiting no signs of bitterness. He blew kisses to the crowd, who responded with a rousing ovation. Vanderlei won the only Olympic medal for Brazil in the 2004 Summer Olympics. He inspired the world. Officials rewarded him with the Pierre de Coubertin medal for sportsmanship, the most prestigious of all Olympic medals [2].

Vanderlei did not lie on the ground and complain about the deranged monk. He called on his own resources and power to successfully manage the situation. I think we often look in the wrong place trying to resolve a difficult interview. It seems natural to first

J. Binder, *Pediatric Interviewing: A Practical, Relationship-Based*   **135**
Approach, Current Clinical Practice, DOI 10.1007/978-1-60761-256-8_10,
© Springer Science+Business Media, LLC 2010

look to the patient and observe what the patient is doing "wrong." We explain the problem by labeling the patient:

"She's a pain."

"She's a bad historian."

"Can you believe the nerve of that mother?"

"He's got an attitude."

We give away our power to influence the interview by focusing on the patient. We could retain our power if only we would focus our attention several feet closer, to our own thoughts and feelings, and use them to help us to influence the course of the interview. This is especially important during challenging interviews. In this chapter, we will examine examples of difficult patients commonly seen in pediatric practice. The difficult interview resembles a difficult clinical situation. When a clinician develops competence recognizing, assessing, and managing difficult interviews, he increases his clinical confidence. A difficult interview provides a wonderful opportunity for the clinician to grow in his competency as an interviewer.

We will examine five cases as prototypal examples. The principles for approaching difficult interviews can be gleaned from these examples:

1. Challenge to a physician's competence. Sometimes this simply presents as a differing idea about diagnosis or treatment. Even when it does not present as a differing idea, such a disagreement is often at the heart of the matter and reframing the challenge as such a difference may help both parties.
2. Families with unrealistic expectations or at least expectations that differ from the physician. What we label as "unrealistic expectations" often are simply differing from ours.
3. Patients or families that the physician experiences as unlikable or even disgusting.
4. Cultural prejudices.
5. Discussing a *problem* in medical care with a fellow trainee.

In previous chapters, we have seen examples of other challenging interviews:

6. Patients who do not describe their symptoms clearly during the HPI (Chap. 3)
7. Suicide and child abuse assessments (Chap. 8)
8. Giving bad news (Chap. 9)

The core skills needed to successfully manage a difficult interview include making effective contact; establishing a contract; tracking with the patient; eliciting patient's thoughts/feelings with the use of gentle commands; taking a slow pace; expressing understanding of the patient's ideas, values, and feelings (empathy); clarifying/summarizing; and negotiating.

CASE #1

Peter, a first year pediatric resident, is evaluating Marie in clinic. The nurse's note lists fever and rash as the chief complaints for this 5-year-old girl. Peter introduces himself as a resident doctor to Marie and her parents. An uncomfortable silence ensues. Peter wonders if the parents are shy or maybe just worried about Marie.

Peter: Tell me what led you to bring Marie in for an appointment?

Mother: To tell you the truth, we thought Marie was going to see a real doctor.

Comment: Peter feels attacked, disrespected, and blindsided. He was not expecting this. He worked hard to become a good resident. He wants to be appreciated. He fires back at mom:

Peter: (sarcastically) You are so in luck. We have real doctors on Tuesdays and Thursdays. Since today is Tuesday you are seeing a real doctor – me.

Comment: Peter reacted defensively. He and the mother, to nobody's surprise ended up with a quite unsatisfactory interaction. Later, Peter considered what went wrong and how he could have responded in a more effective manner.

In his later analysis of the interaction, Peter recognized an early *pivot point* [3]. He had felt anxious and upset after the mother's remark. Peter will be less likely to act out his feelings and attack in the future, if he stays aware of what he is feeling [4]. He could have taken a deep breath and stopped himself from reacting defensively. He might have become curious about what was underlying her remark – in the style of Peter Falk playing Colombo in the TV show. This choice leads down a path of openness and discovery to a positive engagement. Peter could have taken this path if he did not personalize the mother's statement [5]. The truth is: it is not personal. She would have made that remark to any resident.

The statement does not reflect Peter's competence and value. Rather it has to do with the mother's frame of reference.

Peter: Sometimes parents worry that their child will not be properly diagnosed and treated when they see a resident doctor. Is that true for you?

Mother: Yes. I want to make sure nothing serious is missed.

Comment: Peter now has an interview diagnosis. The interview is difficult because the mother expressed her underlying anxiety in a defensive manner.

Peter: Of course. We use a system in which the resident doctor and the supervisory doctor collaborate on the care of each child so we don't miss important information. After I examine Marie, I will discuss her situation with an attending doctor who will also examine Marie. You'll get two heads for the price of one. Is that okay with you?

Mother: Sure.

Peter   Okay, let's get started.

In summary, covert parental anxiety was made overt and then resolved. Anxiety frequently underlies a parent's challenge to a physician's competence. Staying aware of this dynamic allows the clinician to make a thoughtful response to the parent.

One final note: Although humor is a wonderful antidote to anxiety, Peter's attempt at humor came from a resentful, attacking part of himself, which the mother perceived. It fell flat. The mother needed support and information. His second attempt, "two heads" was well received.

CASE #2

Becky Norris is a 23-year-old mother holding her ill baby in one arm, while using her free hand to hold a cell phone. Becky talks to a friend and barely recognizes the entrance of Molly, a second year resident, who patiently waits several minutes before Becky is done with her call. Later in the visit Becky asks Molly to give her medicine for her own cough. Molly is annoyed and aggravated. She takes a time out from the visit and retreats to the resident conference room. She "vents" about the situation to her fellow residents. Her peers understand her frustration. She calms herself down and reenters the room. She finishes her H&P and discusses the baby's diagnosis and treatment with mom. This dialog follows that discussion:

Dr. Molly:	Becky, (Becky said it was okay for Molly to call her by her first name.) *I am having a little difficulty. It seems you and I have different opinions about how an office visit should go.* I would like us to each to give our full attention to each other so that I can best diagnose and treat your baby. You seem to believe that it is okay for interruptions, like cell phone calls. How do you think we can resolve this difference?
Becky:	I had to talk to my friend so that she would pick me up after the doctor's visit.
Dr. Molly:	I hear what you are saying. The problem is I don't think I can practice good medicine if we don't talk about your baby's illness without distractions.
Becky:	I want you to give good care. I am willing to turn off my cell phone.
Dr. Molly:	I appreciate that. There is one more thing. Since I am training in pediatrics, I don't feel qualified or have the professional liability coverage to treat adults. But, I know it would be more convenient for you if I did treat adults.
Becky:	That's okay.
Comment:	Molly understood that she and Becky simply had a difference of viewpoints, an important step to calmly and effectively establish clear boundaries. She did not view herself as victim of Becky or of a dysfunctional medical system. She owned her problem ("I am having a little difficulty") and enlisted Becky's collaboration in solving the problem [6]. We often find that we have different ideas than do our patients or their parents – ideas about the cause of the problem, or the diagnosis, or the treatment, or even how the visit ought to go, as in this case. To resolve those differences, we first have to surface them and look at them together.

Some differences of opinion involve the appropriate management of chronic conditions. For example, parents might believe a child will be cured of a chronic, incurable condition. The physician can use the same approach taken above: own the problem, clarify differences, and negotiate a working contract. By acknowledging and accepting each other's different frame of reference, parents and physician can agree to a contract and to work together despite major differences of opinion.

CASE #3

Ty, an overweight, shy 8-year-old boy in for a checkup, is accompanied by Melissa, his 29-year-old, morbidly obese mother. She seems annoyed. Dr. Smith, Ty's continuity pediatrician, does not look forward to this appointment. He does not enjoy his visits with this family. He feels uneasy about feeling this way, so he brings it up as a topic of discussion during supervision.

Dr. Smith's supervisor asks Dr. Smith what he feels as he enters the exam room that Ty and his mother occupy.

Dr. Smith:	I feel bummed out, uncomfortable.
Supervisor:	Tell me more about this feeling.
Dr. Smith:	To tell you the truth, I don't really want to see this family I feel disgusted.
Supervisor:	Disgusted with whom?
Dr. Smith:	Mother. I know I shouldn't feel this way.
Supervisor:	Where did you learn to think like that?
Dr. Smith:	Well, isn't it wrong to be disgusted by your patients?
Supervisor:	Acting on those feelings would be poor medicine, but the feeling is not bad. In fact, it is fairly common. Many physicians become upset or even disgusted if they believe a parent is not caring properly for her children. Is that true for you?
Dr. Smith:	I think it is terrible for this mother to just let this child become obese and suffer. I know what it is like.
Supervisor:	Holding that belief, no wonder you feel disgusted. I imagine it took courage on your part to acknowledge your feelings.
Dr. Smith:	Yes.
Supervisor:	How might you respond, in a gentle way, to the disgusted part of you, if you were your own supervisor?
Dr. Smith:	I might say it is common to be disgusted with certain patients [7]. Recognizing this would allow the doctor to deal with it and not take those feelings out on the patient.
Supervisor:	Good thinking! In addition, it might be useful to consider what Melissa is experiencing. Possibly, she is imagining that other people are revolted by her,

then withdraws from them, and greets them with a cold demeanor. If you would like to learn more about these dynamics, you might read: *How Doctors Think* by Jerome Groopman. He points out the tendency of doctors to rush through the visit when they are disgusted by patients. This results in diagnostic errors [7]. Do you think there is anything you might have missed with Ty?

Dr. Smith: I rushed through mother's view of the family weight problem.

Supervisor: Let's go check that out.

CASE #4

Sam, a first year resident in the outpatient department, grew up in the Middle East. His next patient, accompanied by both parents, lives in rural West Virginia. Donald, 23 years old, wears a baseball cap backward. He glances away when Sam introduces himself. Jenny, 20 years old, does acknowledge Sam's greeting. She then looks down at her feet for most of the visit. Sam has experienced this type of behavior, a style he calls "stonewalling," previously. He feels his ire rising and his chest is tight; his voice cracks as he talks:

"How can I help you?"

Sam believes this family is rejecting him, possibly because of his heavy accent and Middle Eastern ancestry. Sam does not know what to do. He decides to ignore his hurt, act friendly, and find out the chief complaint. He employs a number of gentle commands in an effort to open up this family, but their responses are terse and clipped. Sam notices the family readily provides information to the faculty member later when she asks them similar questions. This confirms his suspicion that the family harbors a cultural prejudice.

Sam talks with this faculty mentor after the family leaves. She empathizes with Sam's hurt feelings. He then asks her how he could handle the situation differently. She suggests that cultural prejudice, if that is the root of the family's stonewalling, is about this family and not about Sam. If he *knows* that cultural prejudice is about the family and not a statement about him, he can keep an imaginary bubble around himself to protect himself when families *reject* him. If it is about them, their beliefs and expectations, he has options for managing himself in that situation. For example, he could make the situation overt:

"You know, families I see are sometimes surprised they are seeing a doctor from another country. They were expecting to have a West Virginia doctor. Is that true for you?"

Comment: If the family says they did not have those expectations, at least they know Sam is willing to be open and honest. If the family says yes, Sam can use his empathizing and negotiating skills:

Sam: "I imagine it is difficult to expect a West Virginia doctor and end up with a doctor from the Middle East. Do you have questions about my training. I will make every effort to make our communication clear and provide good medical care. That will include talking with my supervising doctor who will also examine your son. We operate as a team. Is that okay with you?"

Comment: Humor might help. When used judiciously, humor can help a family appreciate the clinician's *humanity*.

"It must be surprising to expect Dr. McDreamy and get Dr. Nassif."

Cultural issues are a hot topic. Most medical schools convene periodic workshops covering this vital topic. Learning about the cultures of the patients he will serve might help Sam learn ways of joining with patients from other cultures. He will still need to ask a patient what he thinks and feels, and not make assumptions, in order to understand that individual patient [6].

CASE #5
Noreen, a third year resident, rotating as the senior pediatric resident on a toddler inpatient floor, just finished her first week on the rotation. One of her first year residents (William) sets up a meeting with her to complain about the poor sign-outs of another resident, Claire. Noreen, an astute resident, utilizes the principles she has learned about leadership over the course of her 3 years of residency.

Noreen: William, I'm glad you brought this up. Accurate sign-outs help avoid serious medical errors. It sounds like you feel discomfort talking with Claire directly about sign-out. I think it might help to first set up a meeting of the floor team and make a clear agreement about how feedback – positive and negative – will be handled. I meant to schedule that meeting last week but I forgot. I apologize.

William:	Okay. But, I don't think I can talk to Claire about this situation.
Noreen:	Well, you could. How come you don't talk to her?
William:	I'm afraid her feelings will be hurt and she won't talk to me afterwards.
Noreen:	So, how are you going to deal with your dilemma?
William:	Well, I know good patient care comes first. And, this has already resulted in poor patient care.

Several days later, after the team makes an agreement, William approaches Claire. The team agreed that negative feedback would be better received if: the overall team atmosphere remains positive [4], both parties agree on a time to talk, and any behavior is described without impugning the other person's character.

William:	Claire, I have a difficult issue to discuss with you. Would you be willing to talk about sign-out last Wednesday night?
Claire:	This sounds bad. Is something wrong?
William:	Well, maybe. Claire, when you signed out that night, I know you were busy. You didn't tell me the complete respiratory status of Jeremy Johnson, the four-month-old baby with bronchiolitis in room 208.
Claire:	I told you he was admitted early in the day, was NPO and on I.V. and was receiving several liters of O2.
William:	I know. You didn't tell me about his pulmonary exam, that his respiratory rate was in the 80s, that he was retracting more and that he appeared irritable and tired. I am not blaming you. I had a part in the miscommunication in that I didn't ask for details of his respiratory status either. As you already know, that evening, the nurse called the senior resident to do an emergency intubation. Thankfully, the baby did well. I think we need to do a better sign-out.
Claire:	I agree. I felt rushed but that is no excuse.
William:	I also made an error by not asking for detailed sign-out.

These five cases highlight strategies that are keys to managing difficult interviews competently (Table 10.1). The strategies provide a framework that can be applied to a variety of other challenging situations (e.g., an angry parent; a parent demanding antibiotics for

TABLE 10.1. Keys to challenging patients

Own the problem ("I am having a little difficulty")
Stay aware and manage own feelings/ Do not personalize ("It's not personal")
Clarify different viewpoints regarding roles and guidelines for patient visits
Be curious, not furious (explore patient's underlying feelings/thoughts)[a]
Set appropriate boundaries when necessary

Approach based on Establishing Boundaries in Field Guide to the Difficult
Interview (Platt and Gordon).
[a]Slogan promoted by Ellyn Bader, PhD, and Peter Pearson, PhD.

a viral illness, etc.). In the next chapter, we will discus another type
of challenging interview: patients who wander from topic to topic.

References

1. Selincourt A, Burn AR (1954) Herodotus – The histories. Penguin Classics, New York
2. Vanderlei de Lima. http://en.wikipedia/org/wiki/VanderleideLima. Accessed 25 Aug 2008
3. Shea SC (1998) Psychiatric interviewing: the art of understanding: a practical guide for psychiatrists, psychologists, nurses and other health professionals, 2nd edn. WB Saunders, Philadelphia, PA
4. Stewart I, Joines V (1987) TA today: a new introduction to transactional analysis. Lifespace Publishing, Chapel Hill, NC
5. Bader E, Pearson PT, Schwartz JD (2000) Tell me no lies – How to face the truth and build a loving marriage. Skylight Press, New York
6. Platt FW, Gordon GH (2004) Field guide to the difficult patient interview, 2nd edn. Lippincott Williams & Wilkens, Baltimore, MD
7. Groopman J (2007) How doctors think. Houghton Mifflin Company, New York

11
Wandering Interviews

In the end, doctor and patient have the joint task of constructing a story of the illness on which they both can agree. This is not likely to happen if we don't hear the patient's version first.

Platt and Gordon

The clinician evaluates the interview process itself, especially during the opening phase of the interview. She scans for the possibility of a shut-down or wandering interview. We examined an example of shut-down communication in Chap. 1. This chapter focuses on the other extreme, the wandering interview.

Case: Kelsey, a 4-year-old girl with asthma and cough presents to the clinic with her young mother, Lindsey, and the maternal grandmother, Mrs. Stout, on Monday morning after spending the weekend with her father, Mark, and his girlfriend. We join them several minutes into the interview:

Clinician: So, Kelsey has a runny nose and bad cough. Anything else?

Mother: She feels warm. And, she is irritable. Every time she comes back from her dad's, she is mean. She whines and whines. Nothing will make her happy. She seems overtired. They let her stay up late watching TV with his girlfriend's 3-year-old child. I don't think that is good for kids. I think the kids are a bother to them. I'm the one that calls to arrange the weekend visits. I know it's important for kids to have a dad. He should take better care of her.

J. Binder, *Pediatric Interviewing: A Practical, Relationship-Based Approach,* Current Clinical Practice, DOI 10.1007/978-1-60761-256-8_11, © Springer Science+Business Media, LLC 2010

Grandmother:	I think he is immature. They had Kelsey when they both just got out of high school.
Clinician:	I imagine it is hard to raise a child right out of high school.
Mother:	I think I have done okay. Ben has not grown up
Clinician:	How do you mean?
Mother:	He is more interested in himself than Kelsey. He smokes right in front of her and she has asthma. I tell him not to, but he doesn't listen. He keeps smoking and so does his girlfriend. Would you write a letter telling him it is bad for Kelsey. He makes me so mad. Kelsey...
Clinician:	(*interrupting*) Tell me how long she has been coughing.
Mother:	Ever since I picked her up from her dad's. He didn't tell me when it started. No wonder she gets sick, the way they take care of her.
Clinician:	Did she have the cough when you dropped her off on Friday
Mother:	No. She was perfectly healthy. I wouldn't drop her off if she was sick. She was in a good mood. Her preschool had a Halloween party. Kelsey was all excited talking about it. Kelsey is good talker. She tells me exactly what happens when she goes over to her dad's. I know what she tells me is the truth. She tells me Mark and his girlfriend smoke inside, even though he tells me they go outside.
Clinician:	Oh.
Mother:	I smell the smoke on her clothes when she returns. I send her with her favorite clothes and her blanket. Kelsey likes her routine. She dresses herself mostly.

WANDERING PATIENTS

Wandering refers to the tendency of a parent to talk excessively and move away from the initial topic of discussion [1]. Parental anxiety commonly drives the wandering [1]. Occasionally a cognitive deficit results in wandering and accurate third party information is then needed. Wandering presents a dilemma for the pediatrician [1].

If she lets the parent wander aimlessly, she may not gather all the data she needs to make a thoughtful differential diagnosis. If she cuts the parent off, as did this doctor, she will miss the parent's account of the illness, and rapport may be broken as well. Since this parent's account of the illness constitutes the core of the data needed, the clinician must find a way to listen and ask for essential data not offered by the parent. *This does not mean taking turns*. As we discovered in Chaps. 2 and 3, the clinician must track with the patient and weave in her questions as they develop the narrative of the illness together. Sometimes patients and parents do focus so much on what appears to be irrelevant information that obtaining biomedical data seems impossible. Of course, the parent does not view her story as irrelevant information, nor does she think that she is wandering [2]. When the clinician believes the parent is wandering, she needs a way to structure the interview without losing the parent's story.

Surprisingly little has been written on the subject of wandering in primary care settings. However, clinicians will find a conceptually clear method for structuring wandering interviews in the psychiatric literature. Shawn Shea outlines a gently progressive method to address both tasks of the interviewer noted above. Shea states that physicians sometimes "feed the wanderer" through the use of nonverbal cues, like head nodding, and by continuing to track with the patient as she wanders from topic to topic. Typically, the physician feeds the wanderer from a sense of fear that using structuring techniques will disrupt rapport. More likely, the physician will disrupt rapport only if she acts frustrated and interrupts the patient. Instead, if she adopts a gradual, progressive, structuring approach, the physician will most often maintain a sound engagement [1].

A physician uses the opening phase of the interview to recognize that the interview is wandering. Signs of wandering are: talking fast or profusely; not pausing to allow the interviewer to speak; and moving from one topic to another [1].

MANAGEMENT OF WANDERING

Let the patient tell her story during the opening phase (very seldom more than 5 min). *Wandering patients have the same need to be heard and understood as any other patient. They are not wandering off the topic from their perspective.* It is a mistake to structure the interview too quickly. Let the patient know that she is being heard and understood. If she does not feel heard, she will likely stay anxious and continue to wander or repeat herself as did this parent. In the above interview the clinician could have responded:

Clinician: Lindsey (a clinician can help a patient focus by call-
             ing the patient by his or her name, according to Platt,
             March 2009), let me see if I have heard you right.
             Kelsey came back from your ex-husband's last night
             sick with a cold and cough. She has asthma and you
             pay particular attention to her care so that she doesn't
             get sick. In fact, you are very devoted to her. You are
             frustrated that your ex-husband does not give her the
             same care and that he and his girlfriend smoke, even
             knowing Kelsey has asthma. You have not been able
             to influence him to change. Have I heard you right?

Then, avoid "feeding the wanderer" with head nodding or
other non-verbal cues that encourage the patient to go on [1].
Return to the first topic when the patient wanders [1]. Many
patients respond to this, particularly when taking the history of
present illness during an acute illness.

Clinician: Tell me how long she has been coughing this time.

Mother: Ever since I picked her up from her dad's. He didn't
             tell me when it started. No wonder she gets sick, the
             way they take care of her.

Clinician: I can hear that you have several concerns including
             how her dad doesn't care for her the way you think
             best. It would help me if we could concentrate on the
             cough for now. What you are saying about the care
             by your ex-husband is important. We will return to it
             later. How much has she been coughing?

Comment: Use a concerned tone of voice, not a frustrated tone.
This way the structuring seems like a natural part of the dialog and
rapport remains good [1].

If necessary, further structuring is accomplished by making the
process overt [1].

> "I believe it is important for us to focus on one topic at
> a time so that I can get a clear understanding of Kelsey's
> cough. I hear your concern about the care of your ex-husband
> and I promise we will deal with it later. If we wander away
> from the cough I will bring us back. Is that okay?"

Fred Platt makes one final point. Uncommonly, a clinician must
stop a runaway process through the use of a nonverbal communication, such as touch. Often touching the speaker on a nonvulnerable
spot such as the elbow, plus use of the patient's name will allow
the clinician to stop the talking and intercede to get control of the

process. She might even decide to signal time out. Once the patient slows down, the clinician continues to weave open and closed questions into the dialog [3].

> "Clinicians often believe that they must resort to closed-ended questions in order to control a runaway interview. That is a medical myth. Yes, we need to control the process but we still want to allow the patient or parent the freedom to tell her story." (Platt, March 2009)

Trainees quickly learn and use this progressive method of structuring in their clinical work. We focus on the teaching of trainees in Chap. 12.

References

1. Shea SC (1998) Psychiatric interviewing: the art of understanding: a practical guide for psychiatrists, psychologists, nurses and other health professionals, 2nd edn. WB Saunders, Philadelphia, PA
2. Mishler EG (1984) The discourse of medicine: dialectics of medical interview. Ablex Publishing Corporation, Norwood, NJ
3. Platt FW, Gordon GH (2004) Field guide to the difficult patient interview, 2nd edn. Lippincott Williams & Wilkens, Baltimore, MD

12

Using Experiential Techniques to Teach Interviewing Skills

For the things we have to learn before we can do them,
we learn them by doing them.

Aristotle

PREFACE

Clinicians learn and perform the complex medical skill of interviewing best when they learn it experientially, not just read about it. Learning experientially means practicing the skills, receiving feedback, and using the feedback to improve. In this chapter, I will shift the focus to the topic of teaching, using experiential methods, because of their importance in producing effective clinical interviewers.

Although we know much about the teaching of interview skills, programs to train young clinicians face significant roadblocks in implementing a successful interviewing curriculum. They must develop effective strategies to overcome those obstacles.

ROADBLOCKS

1. Time constraints and medical education focus on disease – the cause, diagnosis, and treatment of disease – rather than on the person surrounding the disease.
2. Strong learner anxiety.
3. Lack of trained faculty.
4. Lack of emphasis, in the medical culture, on the emotional experience of trainees.

J. Binder, *Pediatric Interviewing: A Practical, Relationship-Based* **151**
Approach, Current Clinical Practice, DOI 10.1007/978-1-60761-256-8_12,
© Springer Science+Business Media, LLC 2010

Time

"We don't have enough time to teach interviewing skills."

When faculty members hold this belief, any attempt to teach interviewing becomes easily derailed. Programs that have successfully taught interviewing have the same 24 h in a day available to them as other programs. Some programs prioritize interviewing and teach it well; others discount its importance. No doubt, communication skills are discounted due to the disease or deficit model that has driven medical education for centuries. This emphasis on biological processes persists despite the research (see section "Preface") demonstrating that a biopsychosocial approach is more effective and more humane. Two key ingredients have emerged in successful programs:

- Highly structured teaching of interviewing integrated with other content in the curriculum (see Appendix C)
- Faculty development [1]

Thoughtful integration of teaching interviewing skills with other curriculum content saves time by reducing the need for workshops/seminars devoted to interviewing. Integration presupposes that a core group of faculty have received training to do the teaching [1].

Small Group Role-Plays

Residents frequently develop anxious and avoidant behaviors when they are asked to videotape themselves doing an interview, participate in a role-play, or have their work directly supervised. Commonly, perfectionism underlies this avoidance:

"I'm okay around here as long as I am doing things perfectly or nearly perfectly."

Interviewing "mistakes" are seen as mini-catastrophes, especially when they occur in the presence of peers and mentors. To resolve this problem of avoidance, a learning environment must be established for the resident to feel safe participating, one in which the interviewer does not experience failure. Mentors help establish that type of environment in the following small group, role-play based teaching model.

In keeping with accepted principles of adult education, clear goals and objectives for the role-play are stated. For example, a goal, a broad statement about the purpose of the role-play [2], could be:

"The interviewer will encourage a patient to talk and become activated."

Objectives of the role-play, the means to achieving the goal [2], might include the demonstration of the use of echoing and gentle commands to activate the patient and giving the patient plenty of room to talk. Using specific objectives keeps the work sharp. The teacher emphasizes relevant concepts; the student gains clarity regarding what she is expected to learn. In addition, since the objectives are measurable, everyone can see if the objectives have been accomplished. Preparing the objectives before the session ensures that the teacher is prepared to teach. It also helps the teacher tailor the objectives to his students [2]. The leader can track the progress of the group members throughout the year and adjust the objectives accordingly.

In addition to monitoring the students, good teachers must be knowledgeable, willing to teach, respectful of learners, and communicate concepts clearly. Very good teachers are dynamic and stimulating. Great teachers inspire [2].

Group Leadership
The leader of the small group meets with the group members in a circle so everyone has easy eye contact with any other group member. The leader sees himself as a facilitator, so he does not monopolize the talking [2]. He encourages group members to take charge of their own learning. Typically he talks about one-quarter of the time. Generous use of open-ended questions stimulates thinking. He waits 3–5 s for an answer. If a student responds, he gives her several seconds to elaborate. If he gets no response he rewords the question, gives clues, redirects to others, or gives the answer. He does not embarrass a student or barrage her with too many questions. He listens carefully to student responses. He clarifies and affirms [2]. Since the group consists of only 4–5 members, ample opportunity for students or residents to take a turn role-playing exists. (Residents form groups with residents; students form groups with other students.) I have found that residents and students are willing to experiment with role-plays in groups of this size.

A key advantage of teaching interviewing through role-playing has to do with its **experiential** method. An excellent way to fully understand how to engage a patient, elicit a hidden fear, or set the platform with a suicidal patient is to experience it in role-play. In our seminar, the leader picks a general situation and the resident role-plays the part. That seems more fun than scripted role-plays. And, since role-plays are done without real patients, any number of challenging situations can be scripted. Residents can role-play parents being given bad news or a shut-down adolescent and receive immediate feedback. The role-play is done as realistically as possible in order to simulate real encounters. The resident playing the parent also learns by letting herself experience the parent position ("Be the mom"). In fact, the interviewer and parent can be told to change roles if the interviewer notices difficulty empathizing with the parent [3].

The flexibility of a role-play can be put to good use by any participant. A resident might signal a timeout in the middle and ask for suggestions. One of my favorite ploys as a supervisor involves pausing the interview and externalizing the thoughts of a resident. For example, a resident appears anxious and stuck while assessing a suicidal adolescent. During a timeout in the interview, she worries that she may say the "wrong thing." Another resident then stands next to her and whispers "You may say the wrong thing" as she tries to talk with the adolescent. The interviewer then experiences how hard it is to connect with a patient when she talks to herself like that.

Feedback
Residents not directly involved in the role-play are typically assigned a task such as "Watch how the interviewer joins with a family." This keeps them involved in the group process. In addition, they are accomplishing Bloom's higher order cognitive objectives: application, analysis, and evaluation of the material [2]. After the role-play, observers are invited to give the resident positive feedback. Some residents need to be redirected to tell the interviewer directly what he has done well, instead of telling the faculty member. *That makes it more personal and more powerful*. The faculty member stops the resident if he talks about his mistakes.

Observers offer ***affirmations*** first and then ***options*** for doing it differently. Giving affirmations first helps trainees feel good about what they are doing well and avoids the temptation to focus solely on problem areas. Options are simply another way of interviewing – not a criticism that the resident did it wrong. When the faculty member gives options, it is important to focus on one or two options only, so that the resident is not overwhelmed. The following excerpts are examples of typical role-plays.

Role-Play #1

Goal: Obtain personal story during the opening phase

Objectives: (1) Track with personal story; (2) Use gentle commands
        and echoing

Case: Holly, an 8-year-old girl with recurrent abdominal pain, is accompanied by her mother. Matt, a first year resident, and Holly's mother have agreed on the agenda for the visit. Mary, a second year resident, plays Holly's mother. We join them partway through the opening.

Matt: Mrs. Lincoln, given what you just told me about Holly's abdominal pain, what has it been like for the family?

Mother: What do you mean?

Matt: You know, how has it impacted the family?

Mother: Well. The mornings are real stressful.

Matt: Tell me more.

Mother: Holly has belly cramping every morning. She says she is not able to go to school. I end up being late for work many days. I'm worried that there is something wrong we are missing.

Matt: That does sound stressful. We will talk about that after I examine Holly.

Mother: Okay

Matt: I'm going to ask you more specific questions about the pain now. Okay?

Affirmations given to Matt after the role-play: (Mary, Melissa, Joseph – other residents)

Joseph: You used a gentle command. And, you went at a slow pace.

Melissa: Matt, you did a good job of eliciting mom's worry.

Mary: I felt comfortable talking to you.

Attending: I agree with all the above. You made an effective empathic statement acknowledging Mother's fear. In addition, Matt, I thought you structured the opening well. You did not ask questions about the physical symptom, pain. Instead, you obtained personal information and later let mother know you were going to move to the disease-centered phase of the interview. Do folks have any options? Remember, options are just another way of doing it. No one right way to interview exists.

Melissa:	I might have asked mother what she thought was wrong or being missed.
Matt:	Okay
Attending:	My main option would be to build on the personal story you were gathering. I might have echoed her statement "I'm late for work on many days" and let her talk.
Comment:	Students and residents often need encouragement to persist getting the personal story. This resident was doing a good job gathering the personal story. He just needed to persist in his effort. ***Persistence*** can be helpful in a number of settings. When interviewers ask several gentle commands in a row, they often activate patients who do not say much after the first inquiry [4].

Role-Play # 2

Goal: Expand fully the HPI region of cough

Objectives: (1) Ask about all symptom descriptors

Case: Two-year-old with cough for 3–4 days

Patricia:	(Student interviewer): How frequent is the cough?
Parent:	Real frequent.
Patricia:	Did it wake him last night?
Parent:	Yes, several times.
Patricia:	Is the cough harsh or deep?
Parent:	It's deep and congested.
Patricia:	Has he coughed up anything?
Parent:	No.
Patricia:	Is he running a fever?
Parent:	101 yesterday.
Patricia:	Has he taken anything for the cough?
Parent:	No.
Patricia:	Is he drinking okay?
Parent:	Yes, but he's not eating.

Patricia:	How's he breathing?
Parent:	He's had some problems with his breathing
Patricia:	What do you mean?
Parent:	I had to give him nebulizer treatments last night.
Patricia:	Did they help?
Parent:	For a while.
Patricia:	Did anything else help?
Parent:	No.
Patricia:	How about anything that makes it worse?
Parent:	When he gets active and runs around. He coughs and has more trouble.

Affirmations and then options are given: (Jessica, Matt, Cheri, other students)

Jessica:	You nicely checked to see if the cough was affecting sleep.
Matt:	You clarified what mom meant by trouble breathing.
Cheri:	You didn't interrupt mom. You waited for her to answer before asking the next question.
Attending:	I agree. You asked a number of questions to define the symptom. I really liked your use of an open-ended question to invite mother to describe the breathing difficulty.
Patricia:	I think I asked too many closed-ended questions.
Attending:	Did you take in my affirmation?
Patricia:	No.
Attending:	You might take in the affirmations and feel good about what you are already doing. It is easier to improve if you feel good about what you are doing. We will get to options in a second.
Patricia:	Okay.
Attending:	How about options. Anybody have options?
Cheri:	One option might be to use a gentle command when you first inquire about the quality of the cough, then

	ask if it is harsh or deep if mom doesn't describe the quality.
Patricia:	I like that option. I thought of it after I had already asked mom if the cough was harsh.
Attending:	That fits in with my main option. I think using an open ended statement to start might help you get the data more completely and efficiently. "Tell me everything you have noticed about the baby's illness, everything about the cough and his breathing and anything else you have noticed." Then fill in missing information regarding the descriptors of the symptom by *weaving* between closed-ended and open ended questions, depending on the patient's response. How about doing the interview again with that in mind?
Patricia:	Yeah. I would like to try again.

Repeat Interview

Patricia:	Well, Mrs. Ola, you told me he's got a bothersome cough. Tell me everything you have noticed about the baby's illness, everything about the cough and his breathing and anything else you have noticed?
Parent:	Sure. Let's see. He's had it for a week and it is real frequent. It even wakes him several times at night. It seems deep but he hasn't coughed up anything. I was more worried because he had fever of 101 and isn't eating. I even thought he was having trouble breathing like when he had asthma last year and I gave him a nebulizer treatment.
Patricia:	Wow, that's a pretty complete story. Tell me about his breathing.
Parent:	I could hear a whistling sound this morning when he woke up at 5 A.M. That's when I gave him a treatment.
Patricia:	Have you noticed anything else?
Parent:	Just that running around seems to make him cough more.
Patricia:	I can see how you'd be worried.
Parent:	I am.
Patricia:	Anything else you've noticed?

Parent:	No, that's about it.
Patricia:	Okay. Let's see. When you gave him the neb treatment did it help?
Parent:	Not that I noticed.
Patricia:	I have a few questions. Giving him any other medicines?
Parent:	No
Patricia:	Any other medical problem?
Parent:	No. He's really healthy.
Patricia:	Thank you. You do a great job telling me about his illness.
Parent:	Thank you. You're thorough with your questions. Most doctors don't listen like you do.
Patricia:	Thank you again. I'm going to examine him and then I'll get my attending to come in. Okay?
Parent:	Okay.

Role-Play #3

Goals: Establish a strong engagement

Objectives: (1) Use open-ended questions; (2) Make at least one empathic (reflective) statement.

Case: Jaden is a 5½-year-old boy in for a check-up.

Marian	(resident): Hi. I'm Doctor Miller.
Mother:	I'm Jennifer Lowe;
Marian:	Good to meet you. What would you like to be called.
Mother:	I prefer Jennifer
Marian:	Okay. Please call me Marian. Did you have trouble finding the office.
Mother:	No. The directions were fine
Marian:	Good. What is the main reason for your visit?
Mother:	Jaden has been hyper during the first month of kindergarten. He won't sit in his seat.
Marian:	He won't sit in his seat. Any other concerns?

Mother:	The teacher says he bothers the other kids.
Marian:	That must be worrisome for you?
Mother:	Not really. I think he's just a normal boy.

The interview proceeds for a few minutes then affirmations are given: (Matt, Sam, other residents)

Matt:	I thought you gave a warm introduction. I like the way you clarified how she wants to be addressed.
Sam:	You got a contract for the visit and checked to see if there were any other concerns.
Attending:	I agree. You started with a friendly introduction. Your pace was nice and slow. You gave the mother plenty of room to talk. You attended to mother's feelings. Nice work. How about options. Anybody have options?

None of the group members offers any options. The attending gives the following feedback:

Attending:	Before empathizing with mother you might elicit her feelings:"What has this been like for you?"Wait for her to tell you what she has been experiencing. That way your empathy is attuned to her feelings, and not likely to fall flat. Let's try that.
Marian:	Okay. I'll try it. Jennifer, ready?
Jennifer:	Yeah.

Repeat Interview

Marian:	When you get those reports from his school, what's that like for you?
Jennifer:	Well. I really think he's just a normal boy but the reports worry me a little. That's why I brought him in
Marian:	I see. Mostly you are happy with how he's doing but those reports were a little bit disturbing.
Jennifer:	Yeah.

Role-Play #4

Goals: (1) Perform full assessment of a choking episode; (2) Counsel mother

Objectives: (1) Check parental understanding; (2) Elicit parental feelings

Case: Three-week-old in for clinic visit. We join the resident interviewer halfway through the role-play.

Mother:	The baby choked and turned blue around the lips. He couldn't catch his breath.
Resident:	Wow, that sounds like it would have been scary for you. Tell me about it.
Mother:	It lasted 30–40 seconds. His face turned bright red. It was scary.
Resident:	It sounds scary. What did you do?
Mother:	I picked him up and held him upright.
Resident:	Then what happened
Mother:	After a few seconds he spit up mucous and started to breathe.
Resident:	Where was he and what was he doing right before the episode?
Mother:	It happened right after he fed. He was lying down. I think he might need an apnea monitor.
Resident:	I don't think it is indicated. It sounds like he may have had an episode of reflux of stomach contents into his throat. The gagging was his way of protecting her air passages.

Affirmations are given first from the group members (Mary, Taylor)

Mary:	Even though mom was anxious, you stayed calm.
Taylor:	I thought you kept an even pace and listened
Attending:	You used reflection to empathize with Mom. I think that was important, given mother's scare. I also liked your use of gentle commands to activate mother to tell her story. Does anybody have options?
Mary:	Since mom was so anxious, you might have checked her thinking and then discussed the pros and cons of monitors. Maybe you could first say that a breathing monitor might be helpful but that you want to fully diagnose the problem first.

Attending:	My option piggybacks on that idea. I think it is best to make recommendations only after the evaluation is finished. Provide education and counseling only during the closing part of the interview, not during earlier phases. That will give you and the patient confidence that you have done a thorough evaluation.
Resident:	Okay, but what exactly should I say when she asks for a breathing monitor?
Attending:	What would the rest of you say?
Mary:	You might say, "That's an interesting idea. Let me think about it as we do the exam and try to put this all together."
Taylor:	Yeah. Or you might say, "I'm glad you're working with me to come to a good diagnosis and figure out what to do. Let's get back to the question of a monitor in a bit, okay?
Attending:	Yes. Then much later on you might explain why the monitor isn't indicated here. She'll be more ready to listen to your ideas after she's sure you're heard and understood her ideas. That's sort of a law of conversations, according to Fred Platt (May, 2009): ***Nobody is ready to listen to you until they feel heard and understood.***

Role-Play #5
Sometimes a supervisor offers an option during the interview itself, as when a resident takes a timeout and asks for help. Asking the resident what she is feeling at that moment in time can help her use her feelings and thoughts to guide her.

A first year resident discusses medication use with a mother who gave her child several days of prednisone from the prescription of another child.

Excerpt

Resident:	It is not safe to give children medication that is not prescribed for them.
Mother:	It helped my other child's cough.
Resident:	Children can have bad side effects from medicine.
Mother:	Well, she didn't.

Resident takes a time-out and turns to the faculty member:

"What do you suggest at this point?"

Faculty:	Tell me what you are experiencing.
Resident:	I'm anxious.
Faculty:	What are you telling yourself to make yourself anxious?
Resident:	This mother may really harm her child.
Faculty:	What kind of harm are you picturing?
Resident:	Bad. Maybe, an overwhelming infection.
Faculty:	No wonder you feel anxious. How often does several days of prednisone cause overwhelming infections.
Resident:	Not often.
Doctor: Mom?	When you are anxious how do you respond to
Resident:	Tensely. That's part of the reason she's so tense.
Faculty:	Nice awareness. Given that, do you want to change how you respond to Mom?
Resident:	I don't want to come across as tense. I can just ask her thoughts about giving the prednisone.
Faculty:	Good. Let's try that. Can we rewind and try again?
Resident:	Okay.

Repeat Interview

Resident:	Mrs. Jones, I want to go back to your telling me about giving the baby prednisone.
Mrs. Jones:	Okay
Resident:	Tell me your thoughts about giving the prednisone
Mrs. Jones:	Well it did help his brother, but my sister got on my case. She said I didn't have a medical license and the pills could be harmful. So now I'm a little worried.
Resident:	I can imagine. Well you probably didn't do any real harm but your sister is correct, too. Next time perhaps you could ask our help earlier and hold off the pills until we get together on it.

Mrs. Jones:	Yeah. I could. I'll do that next time. And thanks for not coming down hard on me; my sister thought you would really holler at me.
Resident:	No, I won't. I know you want what is best for your baby
Comment:	Another supervisor might have asked the interviewer to switch roles with the mother in order to understand her position experientially.

Residents experiment with new interviewing behaviors only when they trust that the workshop leader will establish a safe atmosphere, one in which resident "errors" and vulnerabilities are accepted. Several years ago, Amy Edmonson demonstrated that the quality of work in a group is enhanced when mistakes are allowed [5]. A leader who makes mistakes, a leader who does not do everything perfectly sets a wonderful model for the group. Even better is a leader with a good sense of humor, one who obviously enjoys the process. Residents quickly join in the fun. Just watch them role-play a family with a rebellious child. A light-hearted learning atmosphere does not mean a laissez faire attitude about learning. A good teacher makes sure his students learn the material [2]. An individual contract with each student remains an essential component of the curriculum. In a one-to-one relationship, the mentor can address the unique needs of the learner for:

(a) Autonomy – A dependent learner may initially respond more to *coaching*. A more advanced learner would need support for directing his own learning [6]. A student, experiencing success and enjoyment with this individualized support, typically wants to continue learning for a lifetime.

(b) Different learning modalities – A variety of educational techniques allow mentors to match techniques to the student's learning style. In addition to role-play and videotapes, direct supervision using real or simulated patients can be utilized [7]. Rarely, a trainee will panic with one technique (e.g. videotape) and need to use other approaches.

Direct supervision with live patients supplies a practical and flexible tool. A resident works on one or two specific goals. The faculty member sits in for part or all of the visits and gives feedback immediately after the visit. Peers can perform direct supervision and give effective feedback as well. The University of Washington Medical School offers an interviewing elective during which a major part of the supervision is given by peers (per conversation with Larry Mauksch, April 2008). Students take the elective in pairs. Under the guidance of a faculty member, they work as a team interviewing patients and videotaping sessions. They document improvement in interviewing skills during the month rotation via a videotape. Students take turns being the interviewer and the observer. The observer gives feedback on specific skills that are being practiced. In addition, the popular elective saves faculty time. The University of Colorado program uses standardized patients and actors trained to simulate a patient's symptoms, to tell his or her story, and to respond with appropriate affect depending on the techniques used by the student. Such exercises lasting half a day involve four students, four rotating standardized patients, and one faculty member. The students rotate the role of interviewer and during the other student's exercise they serve as coaches, usually watching for specific behaviors and problems that come up during the interview (per conversation with Fred Platt, May 2009).

(c)   Practice – the mentor holds the student ***accountable*** for demonstrating core skills and maintaining these skills over time. (Appendix C provides a sample comprehensive curriculum.)

Faculty Development
Recruiting a critical number of faculty excited about teaching interviewing ensures the quality, homogeneity, and enthusiasm of interview teaching. Mack Lipkin created the well-tested Lipkin Model [8]. The Lipkin faculty development course incorporates teaching-specific skills with reflection by participants on their feelings about teaching and interviewing. Four to five faculty members meet with one leader. Skills are learned and practiced in a workshop for 2½–5 days [8].

The American Academy of Physician and Patient has conducted numerous courses using the Lipkin Model [9]. We can glean highly useful information for faculty development from the success of these courses. Training of faculty generates excitement when small groups are utilized, teaching stems from the learner's needs, and specific interviewing skills are demonstrated and practiced [9]. The training is likely to be successful if clear education goals and expectations are established and contracts are negotiated.

The Institute for Healthcare Communication, headquartered in New Haven, CT, and previously known as the Bayer Institute, has trained over 1,000 faculties in 1-week courses. Many of these faculties now teach in student or resident programs throughout the nation. Their Institute training uses small group exercises with standardized patients and the same model has been used by these faculties in working with residents or students.

Training of a core number of clinical faculty allows for the creation of a comprehensive and integrated interviewing curriculum. A resident interviewing an ill child can be directly observed eliciting a parent's hidden anxiety. Another resident, grappling with a wandering interview in his continuity clinic, can participate in a brief role-play with faculty supervision as he discusses the content of the visit. Comprehensive programs have been received positively by participating residents [7]. Research has demonstrated that interviewing skills can be learned with even brief teaching interventions [10–12]. Modeling is a powerful and often brief intervention.

Whether attending physicians recognize their impact or not, they are modeling patient–physician interactions and professionalism everyday at the bedside. Students and residents observe how they listen and relate to patients. Physicians who interview with empathy and thoroughness are giving a strong message to trainees about how to relate to patients and diagnose medical conditions. Modeling, imbedded in the very structure of teaching outpatient medicine, plays a lesser role on the inpatient wards, nowadays, because of an increased reliance on technology, time constraints, and concerns about patient privacy [2].

Programs can take advantage of learning through modeling by intentionally incorporating bedside rounds into the interviewing curriculum. Some programs focus on the outpatient department. Other programs place value on the outpatient and inpatient teaching of communication skills. They are reinstituting the primacy of inpatient bedside rounds. As William Osler, M.D., noted years ago:

> "Medicine is learned by the bedside and not in the classroom [13]."

Clear guidelines for conducting bedside rounds in both settings protect the patient and support learning of students and house officers. A William Osler performance is unnecessary. Students and residents learn much from the modeling of physicians who give themselves permission to be *regular*. Turner, Palazzo, and Ward make a number of suggestions for sensitively conducting bedside rounds: prepare the team regarding the protocol for the visit; introduce the team to the patient; keep it short and simple; do not use jargon; do not embarrass the student or house officer; and maintain patient dignity and privacy. In addition, the leader decides on learning objects for the rounds and reviews the visit with the team afterward [2] [Table 12.1].

Depleted Clinicians

One feature of modeling is seen in the concept of parallel process. We urge treating our students with the same kindness, compassion, and respect that we wish them to evince in treating their patients. If we are unempathic with our students, it is unlikely that they will be empathic with their patients.

Interviewing programs must face a long medical tradition of discounting the physical and emotional health of medical students and residents. Burned out residents do not perform interviews well. A depleted resident is not fully present to his patients. A clinician must be emotionally present to his patients in order to listen and empathize with them. Training programs, then, must answer the following question:

"How can a curriculum be designed that *teaches* empathy (along with competent data gathering)?" This question takes on increased importance in light of evidence that trainees actually decrease in their ability to listen and emphasize as they progress through medical school and residency [14].

One theory attributes this lack of empathy to the cumulative stresses of medical school and residency: lack of sleep, multiple demands of patient care, education, maintaining relationships at home. This makes intuitive sense; an abundance of data shows a negative correlation between stress, overworking, and performance [1]. The ACGME has recognized this and has taken steps to reduce that stress with a decrease in resident working hours [15].

Many medical educators believe that is not the whole story. Coping strategies help, but only so much. Physician advocates point out that we are in the midst of an epidemic of burnout and loss of meaning among older practicing physicians. One idea receiving a lot of support focuses on the daily losses that physicians experience caring for sick and dying patients. Grief counselors have long been aware of the phenomena of burnout when losses are not acknowledged, validated, and grieved [16]. Physicians have always experienced daily losses taking care of sick patients. Doctors grieve when patients do not get better or die. It is no less painful today than it was a century ago. In addition, physicians, just like all humans, have unresolved losses experienced in their *family-of-origin*. These losses can interfere with present day physician–patient communication. Lipkin et al. found this to be important block to teaching communication skills in their interviewing groups:

"A student who had lost a parent in adolescence found that he could not work with dying patients. Another student with a domineering father encountered authority problems during his patient interviews. Still another student, who craved love, having so little at home, became a compulsive giver, unable to sit limits because she perceived them as inflicting on her patients or teachers the pain she had experienced. Sensitive and supportive discussion of personal issues led to personal and educational breakthroughs and to closeness and trust within the group. Failing to attend to the personal dimensions of learning would have inhibited both personal and professional growth" [8].

Today, in USA, a healthcare system that does not support the primary mission of clinicians – healing the wounded – compounds physician distress. The primary mission of private insurance is to make money. The physician of today must grieve the many additional losses brought on by an adversarial healthcare system.

Losses need to be talked out with friends and colleagues, such as in the Lipkin interviewing group noted above, in order to be resolved and let go. Many physicians stuff their feelings of grief [17]. They have been taught to respond to others, but often do not tend as well to their own feelings. One physician, Rachel Remen, wants to change this mindset. She has written two best sellers: Kitchen Table Wisdom and My Grandfather's Blessing. Her innovative curriculum helping medical students discover meaning in the physician–patient relationship is titled The Healing Arts. This experiential course, adopted by over 50 medical schools, has received positive reviews. Students learn how to deal with loss and how to align their values and hopes with the practice of medicine [18].

When students and residents express and grieve their losses, they free up their emotional energy to be present to their patients. Like the marathoner Vanderlei, they bounce back on their feet and fully experience the connection in their patient–physician relationships. They must continue to monitor their emotional state throughout their careers in order to stay open to their patients (Table 12.1).

TABLE 12.1. Requirements for teaching interviewing skills

Emotional safety
Small groups
Avoid failure
Springs from learner's needs
Individual contract
Clear goals and expectations
Accountability
Skills must be practiced to be maintained
Faculty development – Key for program success

References

1. Novack DH, Volk G, Drossman DA, Lipkin M (1993) Teaching interviewing and interpersonal skills teaching in U.S. Medical Schools. JAMA 269: 2101–2105
2. Turner T, Palazzi DC, Ward MA (2008) The clinician-educator's handbook. Baylor College of Medicine, Houston, TX
3. Cole SA, Bird J, Mance R (1995) Teaching with role-play: a structured approach. In: Lipkin M, Putnam SM, Lazare A (eds) The medical interview: clinical care, education, and research, 2nd edn. Springer, New York
4. Shea SC (1998) Psychiatric interviewing: the art of understanding: a practical guide for psychiatrists, psychologists, nurses and other health professionals, 2nd edn. WB Saunders, Philadelphia, PA
5. Edmonson AC (1996) Learning from mistakes is easier said than done: group and organizational influences on the detection and correction of human error. J Appl Behav Sci 32:5–28
6. Grow GO (1991) Teaching earners to be self-directed. Adult Educ Q Spring 4:125–148
7. Shea SC, Mezzich JE, Bohon S, Zelders A (1989) A comprehensive and individualized psychiatric interviewing training program. Acad Psychiatry 13:61–72
8. Lipkin M, Kaplan C, Clark W, Novak DH (1995) Teaching medical interviewing: the Lipkin model. In: Lipkin M, Putnan S, Lazare A (eds) The medical interview: clinical care, education and research. Springer, New York
9. Gordon GH, Rost K (1995) Evaluating a faculty development course on medical interviewing. In: Lipkin M, Putnam S, Lazure A (eds) The medical interview: clinical care, education, and research. Springer, New York
10. Yedida MJ, Gillespie CC, Kachur E, et al (2003) Effect of communications training on medical student performance. JAMA 290:1157–1165
11. Alexander SC, Keitz SA, Sloane R, Tulsky JA (2006) A controlled trial of a short course to improve resident's communication with patient's at the end of life. Acad Med 81:1008–1012
12. Roter DL, Hall JA, Kern DE, Barker R, Cole KA, Roca RP (1995) Improving physician's interviewing skills and reducing patient's emotional distress: a randomized clinical trial. Arch Intern Med 155:1877–1884
13. Thayer WS (1919) Osler the teacher. Bull Johns Hospkins Hosp 30:198–200
14. Smith AC, Kleinman S (1989) Managing emotions in medical school: students' contacts with the living and the dead. Soc Psychol Q 52:56–69
15. Accreditation Council for Graduate Medical Education. Common Program Requirements. Effective: July 1, 2007 http://www.acqme.org/acWebsite/dutyHours/dh-Com Progr Requirements Duty Hours 07.07. pdf. Accessed 22 Jan 2008
16. Remen RN (2000) My grandfather's blessings. Riverhead, New York
17. Remen RN (1996) Kitchen table wisdom. Riverhead, New York
18. Remen RN The healer's art. http://www.commonweal.org/ishi/programs/healers_art.html. Accessed 22 Jan 2008

13
Glossary of Interviewing Terms

Behavioral incident Specific historical details of a behavior or symptom are asked about in a chronological fashion to obtain valid data and not opinion. Behavioral incidents were described by G. Pascal.

Cannon questions Successive questions asked before the interviewee has a chance to answer the first one, leaving the interviewee unclear about which question to answer.

Checking Interviewer summarizes what she had just heard from the patient to "check" accuracy and/or to give herself time to decide in which direction to go next. (Cole and Bird describe technique in "The Medical Interview").

Circular questioning An interviewing technique developed by Selvini-Palazzoli. The interviewer asks questions based on responses of other family members. How is this member of the family affected by another member's thoughts, feelings, and behaviors. The interviewer can then return to the original family member to complete the "circle."

Contact The level of connection that the interviewer has to the experience of the patient. It can also refer to the extent that the interviewer is in touch with her own thoughts and feelings.

Contract An agreement between two autonomies, people, or parties to a well-defined cause of action.

Echoing back The act of repeating back to the patient what the patient just said as a way of encouraging the patient to say more and of letting the patient know that the doctor has been listening and actually understands what has been said.

Enactment A term from family therapy: Two members of a family or group interact in front of the interviewer. The interviewer assigns a task and then observes the interactions.

J. Binder, *Pediatric Interviewing: A Practical, Relationship-Based Approach*, Current Clinical Practice, DOI 10.1007/978-1-60761-256-8_13, © Springer Science+Business Media, LLC 2010

Engagement The connection between interviewer and interviewee that supports the interviewee becoming activated to talk. Engagement has been called "the grout of the clinical interview" as it fills the gaps between techniques (Carroll G, Platt FW. Engagement: the grout of the clinical encounter. JCOM 1998;5:43–45)

Gates Transition statement joining two different areas of the history. (Shawn Shea describes gates in the *Psychiatric Interviewing: the Act of Understanding*).

> **Implied** Moving to a new topic that is generally related to the previous topic. The transition is *implied* by the similarity of the subject matter.

> **Natural** The interviewer *cues* off a statement made by the interviewee to creatively move to a new topic.

> **Referred** The interviewer moves to a new topic by going back to an earlier statement made by the interviewee.

> **Spontaneous** The interviewee moves to a new topic, often before a topic is fully expanded. The interviewer then faces a pivot point; follow the patient's spontaneous movement to a new topic or return to the original topic.

Gentle assumption The interviewer asks a question assuming the interviewee has a certain thought or is performing a certain behavior. This technique can increase validity (Shea). It should not be used when asking about a history of abuse, since this could lead to false reporting.

Gentle command An open-ended request that often has no question mark attached to it and that starts with:

> Tell me....
> Describe....
> Say something about....

A gentle or caring voice is used.

Hidden agenda An unstated worry of a parent present in at least a third of child illness visits. Of course, calling it "hidden" is a bit of a misnomer. It is only hidden until asked about with inquiries such as "What else can you tell me?" or "What do you worry about when that happens?" Such questions are part of a good interviewer's armamentarium and do not require blaming the patient for hiding something.

Normalization A technique to decrease defensiveness and increase accuracy by acknowledging the universality of feelings or some other human experience. This often decreases the interviewee's sense of shame and isolation.

Personalize   The process of emotionally reacting on the basis of early childhood "decisions" about self and other people rather than the here-and-now reality.

Pivot point   A choice an interviewer has to make between moving with the patient in a new direction or referring back to the previous topic.

Region   The interview stays on a topic for several sentences or more.

Restate   The patient tells the clinician what he heard the clinician say. It is a way to check, recall, and understand. Also called Echoing Back and Short Summary.

Role play   A technique in which a physician/patient interview situation is created and students/residents take the role of the physician and patient/family. Goals for the exercise are established before the start of the interaction.

Safety   An environment that is nurturing, accepting, and nonjudgmental of interviewee's experience. This encourages an interviewee to talk, free from the scare that she will be judged critically.

Third person technique   A normalization technique developed by Michael Rothenberg. The interviewer bypasses interviewee defensiveness by saying "Lots of people in this situation..." He then states what lots of people might feel or think in that situation. He asks if that makes sense to the interviewee and is it true for him.

Tracking   The interviewer attends to the feelings and experience of the interviewee by asking questions or making comments that flow directly from the statements of the interviewee.

Warning shot   A brief statement made before giving bad news so patient and family can prepare themselves.

14
Appendices

APPENDIX A. INCREASING EFFICIENCY WHILE OBTAINING A HISTORY OF PRESENT ILLNESS

1. Listen during the opening phase. Rushing patients can lead to shut-down interviews and missing data. Ultimately time is wasted.
2. Establish an agenda. Find out the chief complaint and any other concerns the family has in order to organize the inquiry.
3. Take symptoms one at a time unless symptoms follow the same chronological course.
4. Start a long review of possible associated symptoms with the following statement: "I am going to review a list of symptoms. Stop me if you have had the symptom."
5. *Guide* the interviewee through the seven cardinal features of any symptoms using transitional statements (gates) or the summarization technique. Follow a set sequence.
6. Avoid the temptation to ask a laundry list of closed-ended questions to get data quickly. Studies show that open-ended questions lead to more information (with a ratio of 2:1) and do it more quickly. It is often most efficient to use open-ended questions to activate the patient and focused questions to fill in missing details. Even then, gentle commands ("Tell me about...") **weaved** into the interview when the patient acknowledges a symptom or problem (e.g., poor sleep) help data collection.
7. *Stay* in one subregion (e.g., the quality or context of a symptom) until it is fully carved out before moving on. If a patient wanders onto unnecessary details, return to the topic using one of the following strategies:

J. Binder, *Pediatric Interviewing: A Practical, Relationship-Based Approach*, Current Clinical Practice, DOI 10.1007/978-1-60761-256-8_14, © Springer Science+Business Media, LLC 2010

(a) Simply return to the original topic area with a question "Tell me more about what the cough sounds like."

(b) Acknowledge family's concerns, then return to the original topic "What you are talking about is important. We will return to it. For now, I need to fully understand the cough and what it sounds like."

8. Move from the general to the specific. In most cases, do not ask specific questions too soon. It can lead to jumping around and losing efficiency.

9. Learn which questions really differentiate conditions by asking experts and reading sources like *The Patient History: An Evidence-Based Approach* by Lawrence Tierney and Mark Henderson.

10. If there is not enough time to deal with one of the problems (e.g., hyperactivity) and it can wait, schedule a return visit.

APPENDIX B. CHRONOLOGICAL ASSESSMENT OF SUICIDAL EVENTS

1. Suicidal events include death wishes, suicidal thoughts, and feelings, in addition to suicidal attempts.

2. Chronological assessment of suicidal events (CASE) is a method of organizing the collection of data in order to avoid the omission of information.

3. The data is gathered in four discrete sections – presenting events (which can be thoughts only), recent events (last 8 weeks), past events, and immediate events (current suicidality).

4. The data is usually gathered in the above order.

5. Validity techniques are utilized throughout the interview, including repeated behavioral incidents and gentle assumption.

6. The use of a behavioral incident with the presenting events helps uncover important data, such as the potential lethality of the event, the intent, how well was event planned, how does patient feel about the event not being successful, the use of alcohol, etc.

7. Corroborative sources are critical.

8. The CASE is a strategy that is easily remembered.

9. It is clearly explained in The Practical Art of Suicide Assessment: A Guide for Mental Health Professionals and Substance Abuse Counselors by Shawn Shea.

APPENDIX C. SAMPLE CURRICULUM FOR TEACHING
INTERVIEWING SKILLS IN A SMALL PROGRAM STRUCTURE

1. *All first-year residents meet weekly in a small group (5–6 members) with a faculty member.* Role-plays are the primary method used for teaching interviewing. Reviewing videotapes of the role-plays are occasionally employed to enhance giving feedback. Each member of the group has an individual contract covering what she will learn and demonstrate over the course of the year. Some of the group time is freed up for brief discussions, questions, and relationship building.

2. All residents attend a monthly seminar on advanced interviewing techniques. A variety of methods are utilized. These include a brief didactics followed by breaking up into small groups and practicing; performing a demonstration interview with a live patient or family; and brief discussions of challenging patients that residents have encountered in their clinical work.

3. All residents have the opportunity to have interviews directly observed in the outpatient department on an ongoing basis. The interviews are directly observed by a faculty member who provides immediate feedback. The faculty member can also demonstrate techniques at the bedside. Residents are encouraged to have peers observe their interviewing directly and give feedback in a similar manner.

Educational content for first-year resident group	Skills
Introductions	Making contact
Activating a patient	Echoing
Obtaining a personal story	Gentle commands
Empathy	Reflection
Nonverbal communication/pacing	Validation/normalization
Smooth transitions	Contracting
Structuring the HPI	Summarizing
Carving out the seven descriptors of a symptom	Eliciting feelings
Open-ended and closed questioning	Natural/referred gates
Closing phase of the interview	Pivot points/spontaneous gates
Asking about underlying fears/self-diagnosis	Third person technique
Talking with families with a chronic condition	Behavioral incident

(Continued)

(Continued)

Educational content for first-year resident group	Skills
Motivational interviewing	Circular questioning
Joining with families	Warning shot
Family conference	Five basic questions
Obtaining a social history	Developing a positive theme
Sensitive topics	Restatement
Suicide assessment	Weaving
Asking about sexuality and substance use	
Child abuse assessment	
Gently structuring a wandering interview	
Opening up a shut-down patient	
Self-awareness	
Giving bad news	
Managing challenging interviews	
Dealing with unrealistic expectations of families	
Clear communication with fellow residents/sign-out,...	
Physician depletion	

APPENDIX D. CAPACITY FOR WELL-CHILD CARE ANTICIPATORY GUIDANCE TOPICS

The Healthy Steps Project developed at Boston University deals with the capacity problem through a team approach utilizing other professionals. It is not unlike the Swedish system of promoting development for all children. A Healthy Steps specialist collaborates with the physician to provide truly comprehensive well-child care. The healthcare specialist provides the family with education, support, and guidance in the office and at home. She may even lead a group discussion for parents [1].

The motivation underlying this type of approach is based on evidence that early childhood experiences profoundly impact *all* children's educational success, as well as their adult physical and mental health [2, 3]. Children raised in welfare homes have heard, on average, 30 million fewer words than children from professional homes by the time they are 3 years old; more importantly, they have received fewer encouraging than discouraging statements [1:2], the exact opposite of children from professional families [6:1] [2]. Disadvantaged children are already far behind when they enter kindergarten. The problem is much bigger than identifying one 4-year-old who needs head start and speech therapy, another 2-year-old who needs physical therapy, etc. If the goal of well-child care is to enhance the emotional, social, and physical lives of all children, rich and poor, advantaged and disadvantaged, then the Healthy Steps and Swedish models fit well.

A second strategy for dealing with the capacity problem is the group visit. Lucy Osborne promoted a group approach in providing well-child care decades ago. Group visits allow for extra time devoted to anticipatory guidance [4]. This is a result of the fact that 4–6 infants or children of the same age are assigned to one long-time slot, typically 1 h. Group visits are *fun and stimulating*. Families interact and support each other. They empower one another. The biggest challenge is the administrative task of scheduling and coordinating visits for families choosing this alternative.

An innovative strategy to help physicians manage one of the important psychosocial issues of families was recently initialized by the Illinois Chapter of the AAP in collaboration with the state of Illinois. A program to screen and treat postpartum women with depression was created. Individual practitioners have financial, educational, and professional support, including access to a single, toll-free number [5]. This approach, integrating physicians with the community, has been shown to be clinically effective in randomized controlled studies [5].

References

1. Zuckerman B, Parker S, Kaplan-Sanoff M, Augustyn M (2004) Healthy steps: a case study of innovation in pediatric practice. Pediatrics 114:820–826
2. Hart B, Risley TR (1995) Meaningful differences in the everyday experiences of young children, 1st edn. Paul H. Brooks Publishing, Baltimore, MD
3. Felitti VJ, Anda RF, Nordenberg D, Williamson DF, Spitz AM, Edwards V, Koss MP, Marks JS (1998) The relationship of adult health status to childhood abuse and household dysfunction. Am J Prev Med 14:245–258
4. Osborn LM, Woolley FR (1981) Use of groups in well child care. Pediatrics 67:701–706
5. Glascoe FP Screening for perinatal depression. http://www.dbpeds.org. Accessed 28 Sep 2006

APPENDIX E. SCREEN FOR CHILD ANXIETY RELATED DISORDERS (SCARED)

Child Version – Pg. 1 of 2 (To be filled out by the CHILD)

Name:

Date:

Directions

Below is a list of sentences that describe how people feel. Read each phrase and decide if it is "Not True or Hardly Ever True" or "Somewhat True or Sometimes True" or "Very True or Often True" for you, for the last 3 months.

0   Not True or Hardly Ever True
1   Somewhat True or Sometimes True
2   Very True or Often True

1. When I feel frightened, it is hard to breathe.
2. I get headaches when I am at school.
3. I don't like to be with people I don't know well.
4. I get scared if I sleep away from home.
5. I worry about other people liking me.
6. When I get frightened, I feel like passing out.
7. I am nervous.
8. I follow my mother or father wherever they go.
9. People tell me that I look nervous.
10. I feel nervous with people I don't know well.
11. I get stomachaches at school.
12. When I get frightened, I feel like I am going crazy.
13. I worry about sleeping alone.
14. I worry about being as good as other kids.
15. When I get frightened, I feel like things are not real.
16. I have nightmares about something bad happening to my parents.
17. I worry about going to school.
18. When I get frightened, my heart beats fast.
19. I get shaky.
20. I have nightmares about something bad happening to me.

Screen for Child Anxiety Related Disorders (SCARED)
Child Version – Pg. 2 of 2 (To be filled out by the CHILD)

0   Not True or Hardly Ever True
1   Somewhat True or Sometimes True
2   Very True or Often True

21. I worry about things working out for me.
22. When I get frightened, I sweat a lot.

23. I am a worrier.
24. I get really frightened for no reason at all.
25. I am afraid to be alone in the house.
26. It is hard for me to talk with people I don't know well.
27. When I get frightened, I feel like I am choking.
28. People tell me that I worry too much.
29. I don't like to be away from my family.
30. I am afraid of having anxiety (or panic) attacks.
31. I worry that something bad might happen to my parents.
32. I feel shy with people I don't know well.
33. I worry about what is going to happen in the future.
34. When I get frightened, I feel like throwing up.
35. I worry about how well I do things.
36. I am scared to go to school.
37. I worry about things that have already happened.
38. When I get frightened, I feel dizzy.
39. I feel nervous when I am with other children or adults and I have to do something while they watch me (for example: read aloud, speak, play a game, play a sport.)
40. I feel nervous when I am going to parties, dances, or any place where there will be people that I don't know well.
41. I am shy.

Scoring:
A total score of ≥25 may indicate the presence of an **Anxiety Disorder**. Scores higher that 30 are more specific.

A score of **7** for items 1, 6, 9, 12, 15, 18, 19, 22, 24, 27, 30, 34, 38 may indicate **Panic Disorder** or **Significant Somatic Symptoms**.

A score of **9** for items 5, 7, 14, 21, 23, 28, 33, 35, 37 may indicate **Generalized Anxiety Disorder**.

A score of **5** for items 4, 8, 13, 16, 20, 25, 29, 31 may indicate **Separation Anxiety Disorder**.

A score of **8** for items 3, 10, 26, 32, 39, 40, 41 may indicate **Social Anxiety Disorder**.

A score of **3** for items 2, 11, 17, 36 may indicate **Significant School Avoidance**.

For children ages 8 to 11, it is recommended that the clinician explain all questions, or have the child answer the questionnaire sitting with an adult in case they have any questions.

Developed by Boris Birmaher, MD, Suneeta Khetarpal, MD, Marlane Cully, MEd, David Brent, MD, and Sandra McKenzie, PhD, Western Psychiatric Institute and Clinic, University of Pittsburgh. (10/95). E-mail: birmaherb@msx.upmc.edu

APPENDIX F. TRANSACTIONAL ANALYSIS ORIGINATED BY ERIC BERNE

Transactional analysis is a theory of personality development, a theory of communication, and a theory of child development. It is a systematic psychotherapy with many practical applications and techniques that help people change. And, it is a philosophical framework for understanding how people *relate* [1]. Three assumptions form the foundation of transactional analysis:

> "People are Okay.
> Everyone has the capacity to think (except those with severe brain damage).
> People decide their own destiny, and these decisions can be changed" [1].

The first statement above refers to a deep conviction about the *essential* worth and dignity of all people. Even though people may behave poorly, their essence remains valuable. Since people are okay and can think, then people take joint responsibility for what occurs in their relationships, including medical relationships. A *contract* that defines the commitment of each individual is a key to a healthy outcome. A second outcome of the assumptions that people are okay and can think is that people should have full information about what is going on the relationship [1]. Finally since people are okay, they deserve affirmations just for existing. Woollams and Brown state that:

> "Positive stoking invites more Okayness and solves more problems than any other type of therapeutic intervention" [2].

For those interested, the first reference listed below is a book that provides a thorough understanding of transactional analysis through self-study.

References
1. Stewart I, Joines V (1987) TA today: a new introduction to transactional analysis. Lifespace Publishing, Chapel Hill, NC
2. Woollams S, Brown M (1979) The total handbook of transactional analysis. Prentice-Hall, Englewood Cliffs, NJ

APPENDIX G. SUGGESTED READINGS

1. *Field Guide to the Difficult Patient Interview* by Fred Platt and Geoffrey Gordon (2004)
2. *Patient-Centered Interviewing; An Evidence-Based Method* by Robert Smith (2002)
3. *The Patient History: Evidence-Based Approach* edited by Lawrence Tierney and Mark Henderson (2005)
4. *Family-Oriented Primary Care* (2nd ed.) by Susan McDaniel, Thomas L. Campbell, Jeri Hepworth, and Alan Lorenz (2005)
5. *Parenting Children with Health Issues* by Foster Cline and Lisa Greene (2007)
6. *Encounters with Children; Pediatric Behavior and Development* by Suzanne Dixon and Martin Stein (2006)
7. *Motivational Interviewing: Preparing People for Change* by William Miller and Stephen Rollnick (2002)
8. *The Practical Art of Suicide Assessment: A Guide for Mental Health Professional and Substance Abuse Counselors by* Shawn Shea (2002)
9. *Lessons of Loss: A Guide to Coping* by Robert Neimeyer (2006)
10. Doctors Talking with Patients/Patients Talking with Doctors by Debra Roter and Judith Hall (2006)

Index

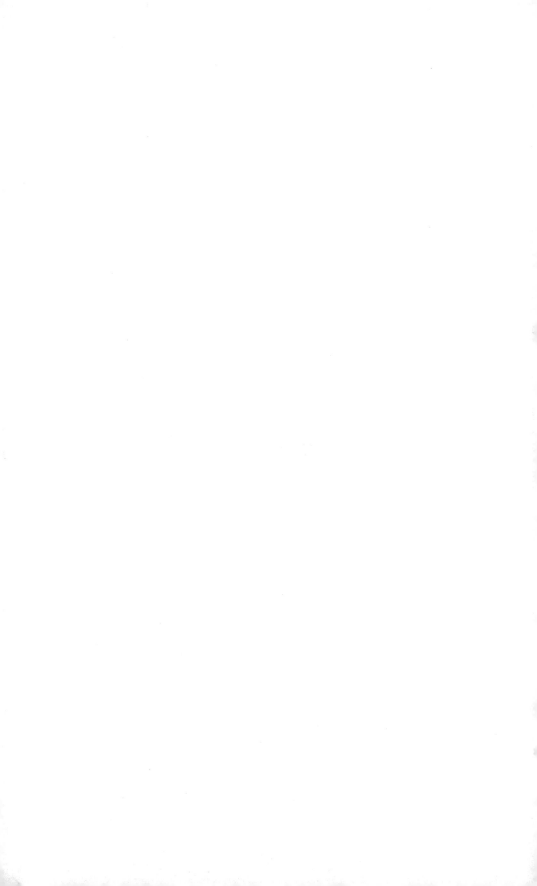